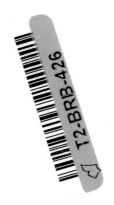

# lunch boxes and snacks

Also by Annabel Karmel

*Complete Party Planner*
*SuperFoods*
*Top 100 Baby Purees*
*Favorite Family Meals*
*The Healthy Baby Meal Planner*


For more information, visit
www.annabelkarmel.com

# lunch boxes and snacks

Over 120 healthy recipes,
from delicious sandwiches and salads
to hot soups and sweet treats

Annabel Karmel

**ATRIA** BOOKS

New York   London   Toronto   Sydney

*This book is dedicated to all those parents who can't face
making yet another peanut butter sandwich, myself included.*

ATRIA BOOKS

A Division of Simon & Schuster, Inc.
1230 Avenue of the Americas
New York, NY 10020

First Atria Books hardcover edition December 2007

ATRIA BOOKS and colophon are trademarks of Simon & Schuster, Inc.

For information about special discounts for bulk purchases, please contact
Simon & Schuster Special Sales at 1-800-456-6798 or business@simonandschuster.com.

Manufactured in the United States of America

3   5   7   9   10   8   6   4   2

Library of Congress Cataloging-in-Publication Data

Karmel, Annabel.
Lunch boxes and snacks : over 120 healthy recipes, from delicious sandwiches and salads to hot soups and sweet treats /
Annabel Karmel.
p.   cm.
Includes index.
1.  Lunch box cookery.   2.  Cookery (Natural foods).   I.  Title.
TX735.K37 2007
641.5'3—dc22                          2007020048

ISBN-13: 978-1-4165-4892-8
ISBN-10:      1-4165-4892-0

# contents

# the creative lunch box

Welcome to *Lunch Boxes and Snacks*, the book aimed at putting the fun back into making packed lunches for children. The ubiquitous sandwich needn't be a slice of ham slammed between two pieces of bread; it can be a delicious, moist filling of chopped ham and tomatoes mixed into cream cheese to fill a pita pocket. Hot meals can warm a hungry tummy on cold winter days, and treats can be made by your child to meet his or her own, sometimes exacting, needs.

According to a recent study, three out of four elementary and middle school parents regularly pack lunches for their children. Packed lunches are typically seen as the healthier option, but this is often wishful thinking. Children are all different, but what they usually want is a quick, tasty meal. A soda, potato chips, and a candy bar can be wolfed down in minutes, saving maximum time for the playground, but obviously this is not an ideal, nutritious lunch that will sustain them until dinnertime. Below are some of the questions that thousands of parents battle with on a daily basis.

- How do you make a packed lunch healthy and still get your child to eat it?

- What do you do if your child is a fussy eater and likes only peanut butter and jelly sandwiches?

- How do you keep the food fresh and still looking good?

- How do you cope when other children bring in lunch boxes filled with potato chips, chocolate cookies, and soft drinks?

- What do you do if you want your child to have a hot meal for lunch when the weather is cold and miserable?

Read on, that's what you do!

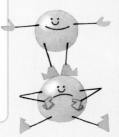

# food for your child's lunch box

In a recent survey on children's packed lunches, it was found that eight in ten packed lunches include potato chips or other salty snacks (see below). More than a third of parents give a chocolate cookie. Healthy foods presented in an enticing way are more likely to appeal to children, like cheese and cherry tomatoes threaded onto a straw, or miniature chicken balls. Both make great finger food.

I'm not a believer in extremes of any kind—I don't think potato chips or chocolate cookies should be totally off-limits to children, but neither do I believe that a jelly sandwich, package of chips, chocolate cookie, and soft drink constitute a proper meal. There is a happy medium, and it's important to remember that habits and food choices begin in childhood and what children eat can make a big difference to their long-term health.

## Top 10 items packed in children's lunch boxes

1 Sandwich  *94 percent*

2 Potato chips or other salty snacks *84 percent*

3 Fruit juice or juice drink  *72 percent*

4 Piece of fresh fruit  *68 percent*

5 Yogurt  *56 percent*

6 Chocolate cookie  *35 percent*

7 Cheese  *31 percent*

8 Chocolate bar  *29 percent*

9 Piece of cake  *26 percent*

10 Cereal bar  *25 percent*

## A healthy lunch box should:

- Help to improve your child's attention span, behavior, and learning in the afternoon

- Provide one-third of your child's daily requirements of nutrients

- Contain a source of protein to keep children alert, complex carbohydrates for slow-release energy, protein and calcium for growth, fat for staying power, and fruit and vegetables for vitamins and minerals

In order to contribute to a healthy, balanced diet, your child's packed lunch should include elements from all the food groups shown below.

## carbohydrates

Choose complex carbohydrates like whole-grain bread, pasta, potatoes, or rice, as they release calories slowly and help to sustain energy levels and concentration. Refined carbohydrates such as white bread, cookies, and cake provide only instant, short-lived energy. Their natural fiber is stripped during processing, and most of their valuable nutrients are lost. The more fiber and protein eaten with starchy or sugary foods, the more slowly those foods are digested and released as sugar into the system.

For fast-release energy, offer banana; dried fruit; apricot; mango; fruit juice; white bread; popcorn.

For slow-release energy, give pasta salad with tuna or chicken; peanut butter sandwich on whole-grain bread; egg sandwich; rice cakes with hummus; pumpkin or sunflower seeds; nuts; raw vegetables and cherry tomatoes; apple; grapes; plums; kiwifruit.

## calcium

Children under the age of five shouldn't have a low-fat diet, so choose whole-milk products like Greek-style yogurt rather than low-fat yogurt. In a recent survey, it was found that 25 percent of young girls were not getting enough calcium in their diet to build strong bones. This could lead to osteoporosis later in life, so make sure that you regularly include dairy products in your child's lunch box. Cheese, yogurt, yogurt drinks, smoothies, and milk shakes are all excellent sources of calcium.

## fruit and vegetables

Health experts recommend that we try to include five portions of fruit and vegetables in our diet every day. To give you an idea of what counts as one portion, here are some examples:

- 1 medium-size piece of fruit such as an apple or banana
- A small bunch of grapes, 2 small fruits (for example, apricots), or a cupful of berries
- ¼ cup dried fruit
- 1 serving of salad or fruit salad
- ½ cup cooked or raw vegetables
- 1 glass of fruit juice or fruit smoothie

Some fruits and vegetables provide different vitamins and minerals than others, so try to offer a wide variety. It's a good idea to include a vitamin C–rich drink like orange juice or cranberry juice to help boost iron absorption. Choose unsweetened fruit juices or nutritious fruit smoothies. Dried fruits are also full of goodness. Raw vegetables with a dip and salads with a tasty dressing are popular ways to get children to eat more vegetables.

## protein

Some good sources of protein are chicken, tuna, eggs, cheese, and peanut butter. These can be used to make delicious sandwiches, pita pockets, and tortilla wraps. You can also make great pasta, rice, or couscous salads with meat, chicken, fish, or beans.

**fat**

Young children require more fat in their diet than do adults, but this should come mainly from nutritious foods like cheese, avocado, and nuts.

## packing your child's lunch box

- When choosing a lunch box, make sure that it is big enough to hold all the food your child needs, but not so large that the food rattles around and your child has an unnecessarily bulky bag to carry. It's a good idea to select a box that is insulated and will accommodate an ice pack to keep food fresh. Make sure you put your child's name on the lunch box.

- Keep on hand some small plastic containers that will fit in your child's lunch box. This will enable you to keep different foods separate—very useful for sandwiches, homemade salads, and ready-prepared fresh fruit.

- There's nothing more stressful than trying to do too much in the morning and worrying that your child will be late for school. So it's a good idea to set out things like lunch boxes, plastic containers, napkins, and utensils the night before. Pack up what you can—like muffins, cookies, and fruit—and make a list of the food you need to make and pack in the morning.

- Keep a good supply of plastic wrap, foil, twist ties, and sandwich bags.

- It's worth buying a wide-mouthed thermos for storing hot soup or pasta.

- Cutlery widens the range of foods you can put in your child's lunch box. Why not get some colorful plastic knives, forks, and spoons?

- Ensure that lids are tight fitting and screw on well, but also check that your child can open them.

- Chopped-up vegetables like carrot sticks can dry out. This can be prevented by wrapping them in damp paper towels.

- Most salad dressings are best packed separately in small plastic containers; otherwise salads can become quite soggy and limp.

- Next time you are in a fast-food restaurant, save mini portions of ketchup, salad dressing, and other sauces. They are always useful for lunch boxes.

## snacks

Snacks are vital for children to maintain their energy between meals. It's important to choose foods that are healthy, as children often eat more between meals than they do at mealtimes.

That said, there is no need to ban unhealthy snacks entirely. The occasional slice of chocolate cake or bag of potato chips won't hurt. Depriving your child of these foods will only make them more desirable.

## safety

- Think of all the foods that we commonly keep in the fridge. Those are the ones that can spoil between the time your child leaves the house and the time she eats her lunch. Try to ensure they are kept cool.

- You can make sandwiches on frozen bread. The cold bread will help to keep the rest of the lunch box cool, and the bread will have thawed by lunchtime.

- An insulated lunch box will guard against the breeding of germs if the box is left in a warm place. To keep your child's lunch box cool, buy a mini ice pack or freezer gel pack, which can be frozen and inserted with the lunch. Buy a couple of ice packs so that you will always have one in the freezer. Alternatively, freeze a carton or plastic bottle of juice overnight. The frozen drink will help to keep food cool and it will have thawed by lunchtime.

- Test the efficiency of your child's thermos to make sure it keeps food hot or cold. Some of those that come with lunch boxes aren't very effective.

- If a child has a serious allergy to peanuts, the school may insist that no children in the class be allowed to bring products containing peanuts in their lunch boxes.

- It is a good idea to pack a small package of wet wipes in the lunch box so that your child can clean her hands.

## getting children involved

- Take your child with you sometimes when you shop for food. If this isn't convenient, get her to make a list of foods that she would like you to buy.

- Try brainstorming some lunch box and snack ideas with your child, and plan her lunch boxes two or three days ahead. Perhaps let your child look through this book and pick out a few new recipes to try each week.

- If you have the time, your child can help prepare some of the food that goes into her lunch box. She could help make her own sandwiches or salads, or on the weekend, you could make muffins, cookies, or Rice Krispies Treats together.

- Invest in some cookie cutters; there are some wonderful shapes to be found. Your child will enjoy cutting sandwiches into novelty shapes.

## something hot

As the colder weather sets in, it's a good idea to include something hot in a lunch box. A wide-mouthed mini thermos would be ideal for serving up a delicious cup of homemade or store-bought soup such as tomato, vegetable, chicken noodle, or minestrone. Other good ideas for hot food that you can put in a thermos are:

- Vegetable stir-fry with noodles
- Bolognese sauce with pasta
- Chili con carne
- Stir-fried rice with chicken

# encouraging your child to eat

Nutrition is important, but let's face it, it's parents rather than children who are concerned about the healthy aspect of food. However healthy the food is, your child won't eat it unless she finds it tasty and appealing.

When your child takes her lunch to school, she carries a little piece of home with her. When my three children had to take in lunch boxes, it became a challenge to come up with something new to entice them to eat healthy food and bring a smile to their faces after a long morning. Simple touches can make all the difference. Try cutting sandwiches into shapes using cookie cutters, or threading fruit onto a straw to make fresh-fruit skewers.

Variety is the spice of life, and with a little effort, there can be so much more to lunch boxes than sandwiches, chips, and chocolate cookies. With this book, I aim to give you lots of choices, ideas, and inspiration to make really special lunch boxes for your children to enjoy as they grow up—without your spending long hours in the kitchen. You will find plenty of enticing recipes on the following pages.

## Small additions make life more interesting

There are some popular mini snacks now available in supermarkets that are ideal for lunch boxes. Here are some ideas for you to try:

- String cheese
- Miniature cheeses
- Twin cartons of cream cheese with miniature breadsticks
- Probiotic mini yogurt drinks
- Mini packs of dried fruit or nuts and raisins
- Vegetable chips made from carrot, sweet potato, and beets

- Cereal and dried-fruit bars (choose ones that are not loaded with sugar or fat)
- Yogurt-covered raisins
- Individual portions of fruit puree, such as apple, or apple and strawberry
- Nuts, if there is no family history of nut allergy; honey-roasted cashew nuts are delicious
- Dried fruit, such as apricots, figs, apples, or raisins
- Pita bread with hummus
- Rice cakes or breadsticks
- Home-popped popcorn
- Wheat crackers

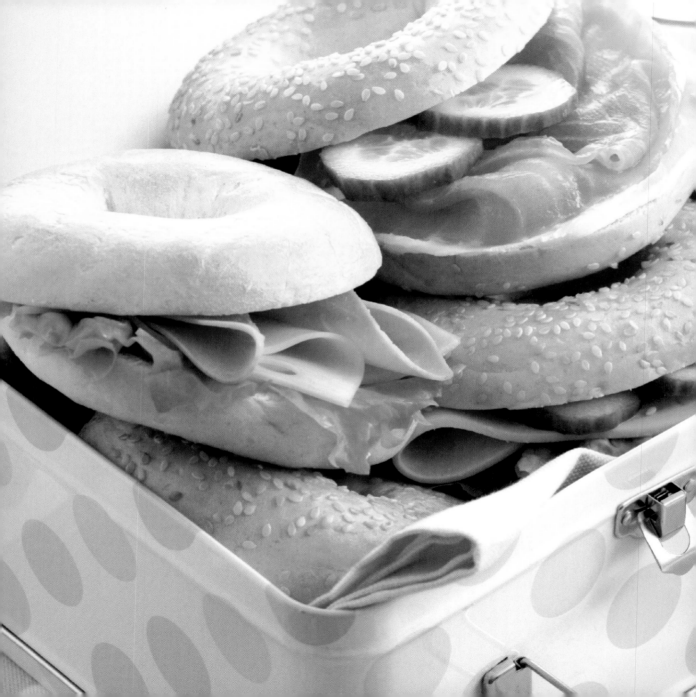

# special sandwiches

Sandwiches don't have to be boring—try novelty-shaped cutout sandwiches, double-decker sandwiches, pita pockets, or tortilla wraps.

*smoked salmon and cream cheese bagel (see page 21)*

# the perfect sandwich

**There are so many different types of breads available now in the supermarket that can be used to make sandwiches. Try ciabatta, multi-grain or whole wheat bread, mini pita pockets, mini baguettes, raisin bread, bagels, rye or 7- or 12-grain bread.**

If you are usually in a rush in the morning, it will help if you get the ingredients together and make up your tuna or egg salad the night before.

To keep the sandwiches fresh, always wrap in plastic wrap or foil as soon as you have made them.

To prevent sandwiches from getting squashed, store them in a small plastic container in your child's lunch box.

Start a cookie cutter collection. Cutting a sandwich into a fun shape like a teddy bear, heart, or car makes it much more exciting to eat. Older children will love to cut out the shapes themselves.

Keep a selection of breads in the freezer for emergencies. You can take out two slices of frozen bread in the morning to make a sandwich. It will thaw by lunchtime and is less likely to absorb the filling.

To avoid soggy sandwiches, make sure you use dry ingredients. It's important to wash lettuce, but dry it before putting it into the sandwich. It may also be an idea to pack wet ingredients separately. For example, sliced tomato can seep into bread, so either pack it separately and let your child add it to her sandwich or put a layer of washed and dried lettuce on top of the tomato.

You can encourage your child to eat whole wheat bread by making "mismatch" sandwiches from one slice of whole wheat bread and one slice of white.

## favorite sandwich fillings

- Cream cheese and . . .
  cucumber; chives; smoked salmon; crushed pineapple; chopped dried apricots; raisins; banana with a squeeze of lemon and honey

- Tuna and . . .
  corn; scallion and mayonnaise; diced celery or cucumber and mayonnaise; chopped egg and mayonnaise; avocado and mayonnaise with a squeeze of lemon juice

- Peanut butter and . . .
  sliced banana with or without honey; strawberry jam or grape jelly; raisins; grated carrot; diced apple

- Grated cheese and carrot with mayonnaise

- Chopped hard-boiled egg mixed with mayonnaise, a pat of butter or margarine, snipped chives or alfalfa sprouts, salt and pepper

- Sliced Swiss cheese, cherry tomatoes, and shredded lettuce

- Grated Cheddar and relish

- Hummus mixed with grated carrot and thinly sliced cucumber
- Hummus, diced tomato, and chopped hard-boiled egg
- Mashed sardines with ketchup and thinly sliced cucumber
- Canned or fresh salmon with mayonnaise, ketchup, and cucumber or scallion
- Shredded chicken, chopped tomato, chopped hard-boiled egg, chives, lettuce, and mayonnaise
- Roast chicken, corn, and mayonnaise
- Mayonnaise mixed with a little pesto tossed with shredded chicken and lettuce
- Sliced turkey or ham, Swiss cheese, tomato, cucumber, and alfalfa sprouts with a little mayonnaise
- Roast beef, lettuce, pickle slices, tomato, and a little mild horseradish or mustard
- Ham, diced pineapple, and cottage cheese
- Bacon, lettuce, tomato, and mayonnaise
- Coronation Chicken (see page 16)

## to help you on your way

- Keep a supply of bread, rolls, bagels, pita bread, and so on in the freezer for emergencies.

## it's a wrap

Wraps are the new trendy sandwich.

- Keep leftover roast, grilled, or barbecued chicken.
- Spread the tortilla with a little mayonnaise and fill with combinations like slices of grilled chicken with strips of tomato and shredded lettuce, or shredded cooked chicken mixed with corn, sprouts, scallions, and mayonnaise.

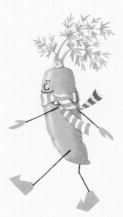

# quick and yummy sandwich fillings

## coronation chicken

Coronation Chicken has a delicious flavor and will keep for several days in the fridge. It makes a great sandwich filling with some crisp lettuce between the slices of bread or rolled up inside a mini tortilla or in a pita pocket. Coronation Chicken can also be served as a salad with rice, popped into a plastic container, and packed up with the rest of the lunch.

▽ **Makes 4 portions**
½ chicken bouillon cube, dissolved in 1 cup
    boiling water, or 1 cup chicken broth
1 bay leaf
2 small skinless, boneless chicken breasts,
    cut into bite-size chunks
1 tablespoon vegetable oil
1 small onion, finely chopped
1 teaspoon medium curry powder
1½ tablespoons mango chutney
1½ tablespoons lemon juice
1½ teaspoons tomato paste
½ cup mayonnaise
⅓ cup plain yogurt
fruit, such as seedless grapes or chopped
    mango (optional)

Put the dissolved bouillon into a saucepan together with the bay leaf. Bring to a boil, then reduce the heat and poach the chicken for about 6 minutes. Leave the chicken in the bouillon to cool down.

Heat the oil in another saucepan, add the onion, and sauté for 2 minutes. Stir in the curry powder and cook for 30 seconds. Stir in the mango chutney, lemon juice, tomato paste, and ½ cup of the bouillon. Simmer for 10 minutes. Strain through a sieve and allow to cool.

Mix together with the mayonnaise and the yogurt, then combine with the chicken and fruit (if using) and chill for a couple of hours or overnight.

## shrimp and arugula with tomato mayonnaise

▽ **Makes 2 portions**
4 slices whole-grain bread
softened butter or margarine
handful of arugula, trimmed and chopped
½ cup small peeled cooked shrimp
2 tablespoons mayonnaise
1 tablespoon ketchup
1 tomato, seeded and diced (optional)
paprika (optional)

Spread two slices of the bread with butter or margarine and arrange the arugula on the bread. Mix the shrimp together with the mayonnaise and ketchup, mix in the tomato (if using), and spoon onto the arugula. Sprinkle with a little paprika if you wish. Sandwich together with the remaining bread, cut into quarters, and trim the crusts.

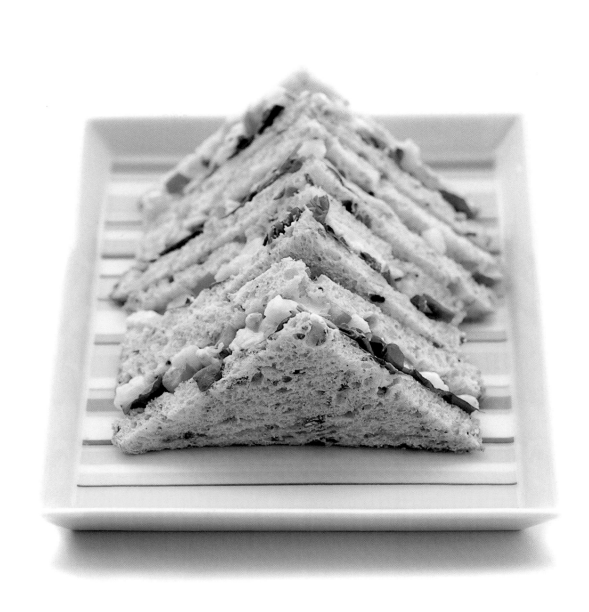

## tuna and tomato mayonnaise

◯ **Makes 1 portion**
*half a 6-ounce can tuna (or salmon), drained*
*1 teaspoon softened butter or margarine*
*1 tablespoon ketchup*
*1 tablespoon mayonnaise*
*¼ cup diced cucumber*
*1 scallion, finely sliced*

Flake the tuna with a fork. Add the butter
or margarine, ketchup, and mayonnaise
and stir in the cucumber and scallion.

## classic blt

There is something completely addictive about
the combination of bacon, lettuce, and tomato—
a classic sandwich filling indeed.

◯ **Makes 1 portion**
*4 slices bacon*
*crisp lettuce leaves*
*2 slices whole-grain bread, buttered*
*1 small tomato, sliced*
*mayonnaise*

Broil the bacon until well cooked. Lay the lettuce
leaves over one slice of the bread, cover with
the sliced tomato, and add a little mayonnaise.
Chop the bacon and scatter evenly over the
tomato. Cover the bacon with the remaining
slice of bread. Press together gently and cut
into two triangles.

## roast beef

Roast beef on rye bread makes a good combination,
and with some small additions like lettuce and
horseradish, it becomes an even better sandwich.

◯ **Makes 1 portion**
*2 crisp lettuce leaves*
*2 slices rye bread, buttered*
*2 slices rare lean roast beef*
*prepared horseradish or mustard*
*pickle slices*

Lay the lettuce over one slice of the bread and
cover with the roast beef, a little horseradish or
mustard, and a few slices of pickle. Cover with the
remaining slice of bread and cut into two triangles.

## pastrami on rye

◯ **Makes 1 portion**
*1 tablespoon mayonnaise*
*¼ teaspoon honey*
*pea-size dot of Dijon mustard*
*freshly ground black pepper*
*2 slices rye bread*
*4 thin slices pastrami*
*small handful of shredded arugula or Bibb lettuce*

Mix the mayonnaise, honey, and mustard together
and season with black pepper. Spread over the rye
bread. Lay the pastrami over one slice of the bread.
Scatter the arugula or Bibb lettuce on top and cover
with the remaining slice of bread. Cut in half.

# chicken and egg double-decker

◯ Makes 1 portion

**Egg mayonnaise**
*1 hard-boiled egg*
*½ teaspoon soft margarine*
*1½ teaspoons mayonnaise*
*2 tablespoons shredded lettuce*
*pinch of paprika*
*salt and freshly ground black pepper*

*2 slices white bread, buttered on one side*
*1 slice whole wheat bread, buttered on both sides*

**Chicken and tomato**
*4 thin slices tomato*
*¼ cup cooked and shredded chicken*
*1 teaspoon mayonnaise*

To make the egg mayonnaise, chop the hard-boiled egg and mix together with the margarine and mayonnaise. Stir in the lettuce and sprinkle with paprika and seasonings.

Cover one slice of the white bread with the egg mayonnaise and top with the whole wheat bread.

To make the chicken filling, arrange the tomato slices on top of the whole wheat bread. Mix the chicken with the mayonnaise, spread over the tomato, and top with the remaining slice of white bread.

With a sharp knife, trim off the crusts and cut into three strips.

**Other double-decker fillings to try:**

- Mashed sardines with ketchup/cream cheese and cucumber
- Chopped hard-boiled egg with mayonnaise, corn, and scallion
- Smoked salmon/cream cheese and chives
- Ham/sliced cheese and relish
- Ham/ricotta with apricots and honey (see page 20)
- Peanut butter and sliced banana/strawberry jam

## grilled turkey and cheese sandwich

◯ **Makes 2 portions**

*4 slices bread, buttered*
*4 slices provolone or mozzarella cheese*
*¼ cup marinara sauce*
*1½ tablespoons freshly grated Parmesan cheese*
*4 thin slices deli roast turkey*

Heat a nonstick skillet or griddle to medium heat. Take two slices of the bread, turn them butter side down, and place a slice of provolone or mozzarella on top of each. Spread with 1 to 2 tablespoons of marinara sauce, sprinkle some Parmesan on top, and add a layer of turkey and another slice of provolone or mozzarella. Top with the remaining slices of bread, butter side up.

Place the sandwiches in the hot frying pan or on the griddle and cook for about 2 minutes on each side until golden brown and the cheese has melted. Slice in half diagonally and serve warm. These can also be made in an electric sandwich maker.

## ricotta with apricots and honey

◯ **Makes 2 portions**

*⅓ cup ricotta cheese*
*1 teaspoon honey*
*3 dried apricots, chopped*
*4 slices bread*

Mix together the ricotta and honey and stir in the chopped apricots. Spread on two slices of the bread, top with the remaining slices, and cut in half.

## turkey, muenster, and cranberry sandwich

◯ **Makes 1 portion**

*3 thin slices deli roast turkey*
*1 small slice Muenster cheese*
*2 slices whole-grain bread, buttered*
*1 tablespoon mayonnaise*
*2 teaspoons chopped dried cranberries*
*1 teaspoon finely sliced scallion*
*salt and freshly ground black pepper*
*small handful of shredded lettuce*

Lay the turkey and cheese on one slice of the bread. Mix together the mayonnaise, cranberries, scallion, and seasonings. Spread over the cheese, then scatter the lettuce on top. Add the second slice of bread and cut into four pieces.

## ham and cheese sandwich

◯ **Makes 1 portion**

*1 large, thin slice Swiss cheese*
*1 slice smoked ham (or turkey)*
*2 slices tomato*
*4 thin slices cucumber*
*2 slices bread, buttered*
*salt and freshly ground black pepper*
*mayonnaise*

Place the cheese, ham, tomato, and cucumber on one slice of the bread and season. Spread mayonnaise on the second slice of bread, then place on top of the filling. Trim off the crusts with a sharp knife and cut into two triangles.

# club sandwich

⬭ **Makes 1 portion**
*few crisp lettuce leaves*
*2 slices whole wheat bread, buttered*
*2 slices cooked chicken breast*
*2 slices crispy bacon*
*2 slices tomato*
*mayonnaise*

Place some of the lettuce on one slice of the bread. Arrange the chicken, bacon, and tomato on top, and add a little mayonnaise. Cover with some lettuce and, finally, the other slice of bread. Cut the sandwich in half.

# bagel fillings

**Omega-3's are especially good brain boosters and can be of benefit to hyperactive children. Smoked salmon is rich in omega-3's. The smoked salmon and cream cheese mix is also yummy on a baguette (see page 23). Try some of these fillings:**

• Diced ham or chicken with chopped pineapple chunks and mayonnaise

• Chopped hard-boiled egg and mayonnaise mixed with a little sweet pickle relish

• Sliced turkey, Swiss cheese, tomato, lettuce, and salad dressing or mayonnaise

# chicken and sun-dried tomato

⬭ **Makes 1 portion**
*1 tablespoon cream cheese*
*½ teaspoon red pesto*
*1 sun-dried tomato in oil, drained and chopped*
*2 tablespoons chopped cooked chicken (or turkey)*
*1 bagel*
*some shredded lettuce*

Mix together the cream cheese and pesto and stir in the tomato and chicken. Slice the bagel in half horizontally, spread the base with the cream cheese and chicken mix, add some shredded lettuce, and top with the lid of the bagel.

# smoked salmon and cream cheese

⬭ **Makes 1 portion**
*1 bagel*
*2 tablespoons cream cheese*
*1 teaspoon snipped fresh chives*
*few slices cucumber (optional)*
*sliced smoked salmon*
*squeeze of lemon juice*
*freshly ground black pepper (optional)*

Slice the bagel in half horizontally. Mix together the cream cheese and chives and spread over the base of the bagel. Lay the cucumber (if using) and smoked salmon on top and squeeze a little lemon juice over it. Finish with a grinding of black pepper (if using).

*(see photograph on pages 12–13)*

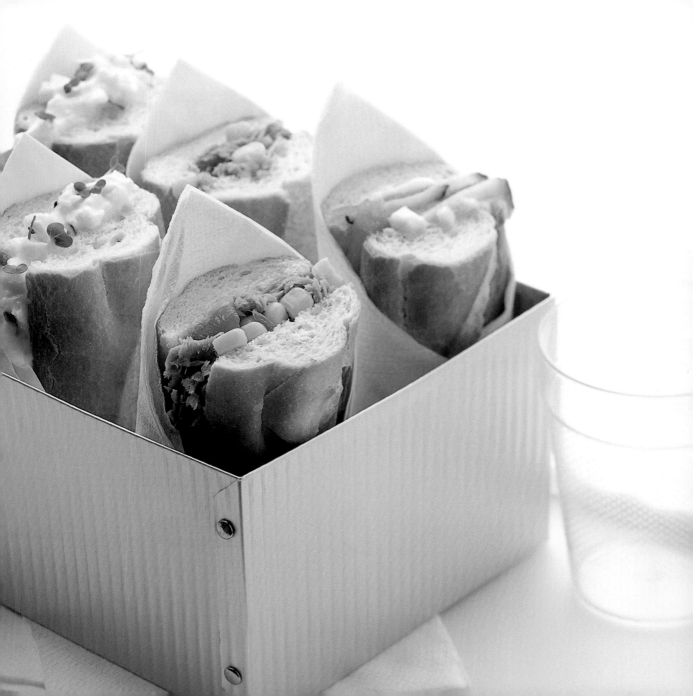

# baguette fillings

**Mini baguettes are popular and can be used with either savory or sweet fillings. Here are my favorites, which are all quick to make and are therefore ideal for when you're coping with that morning rush! They are also great fillings for sandwiches. The tuna mix is perfect in pita bread or spread onto a tortilla, which is then rolled up and wrapped with foil or plastic wrap.**

## tuna with tomatoes and corn

▽ **Makes 1 portion**

*one 6-ounce can tuna in oil, drained*
*2 tablespoons mayonnaise*
*1 tablespoon ketchup*
*2 sun-dried tomatoes in oil, chopped (optional)*
*1 scallion, finely sliced*
*2 tablespoons corn*

Flake the tuna with a fork and mix together with the mayonnaise and ketchup. Stir in the tomatoes (if using), scallion, and corn.

---

**TOP SNACKING TIPS**

Stock up with healthy snacks and plan ahead so that you're not forced to give your children sugary foods when they need refueling after school.

---

## egg and alfalfa sprouts

▽ **Makes 1 portion**

*2 eggs*
*2 tablespoons mayonnaise*
*pat of softened butter or margarine*
*salt and freshly ground black pepper*
*handful of alfalfa sprouts*

Put the eggs in a saucepan of cold water and bring to a boil. Reduce the heat and simmer for 7 to 8 minutes. Drain the eggs and cool them under cold water. When they are cold, peel off the shells. Chop the eggs and put in a bowl together with the mayonnaise, butter or margarine, and salt and pepper and mix well. Finally, stir in the alfalfa sprouts.

## peanut butter, jelly, and banana

▽ **Makes 1 portion**

*1 mini baguette*
*1 heaping tablespoon peanut butter*
*1 tablespoon grape jelly or strawberry or*
  *raspberry jam*
*1 small banana, sliced*

Slice the baguette in half lengthwise. Spread the peanut butter over one side of the baguette. Spread the jelly or jam over the peanut butter and top with the sliced banana.

# annabel's italian sub

◯ **Makes 1 portion**
1 tablespoon mayonnaise
1 teaspoon freshly grated Parmesan cheese
pinch of Italian seasoning (optional)
1 hot dog bun, split lengthwise
2 slices salami
½ slice provolone cheese
2 thin slices deli ham
small handful of shredded lettuce

Mix together the mayonnaise, Parmesan, and Italian seasoning (if using). Spread the mixture over both halves of the hot dog bun. On the bottom half of the bun, lay the salami, provolone, and ham, scatter the lettuce on top, then cover with the other half of the bun.

# annabel's american hero

◯ **Makes 1 portion**
1 tablespoon mayonnaise
pea-size dot of Dijon mustard (or to taste)
salt and freshly ground black pepper
1 hot dog bun, split lengthwise
2 thin slices deli ham
1 small slice Cheddar cheese
2 thin slices deli honey-roast turkey
2 or 3 thin slices tomato
small handful of shredded lettuce

Mix together the mayonnaise, Dijon mustard, and salt and pepper. Spread the mixture over both halves of the hot dog bun. On the bottom half of the bun, lay the ham, cheese, and turkey, followed by the tomato. Scatter the lettuce on top and cover with the other half of the bun.

> **LUNCH BOX LOWDOWN**
> If your child likes potato chips but you don't want him to fill himself up by eating a whole package, put some in a small bag and tie the top, or wrap some in foil.

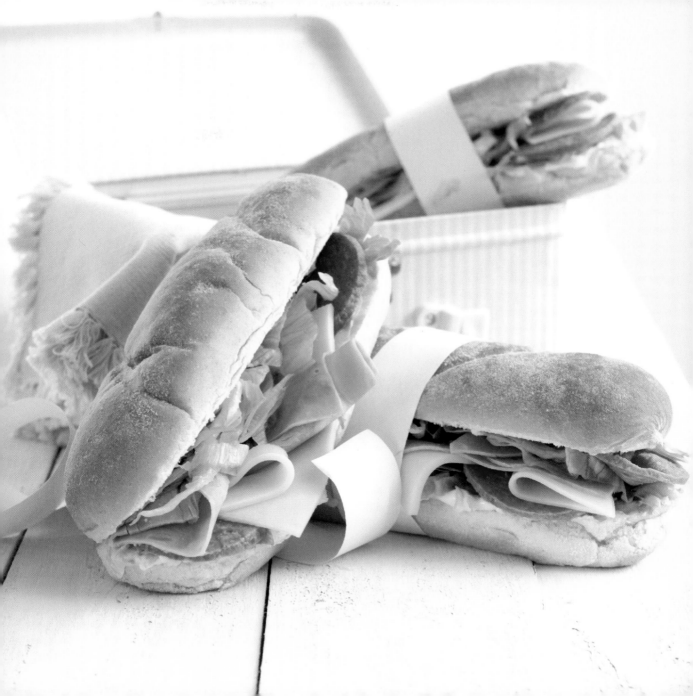

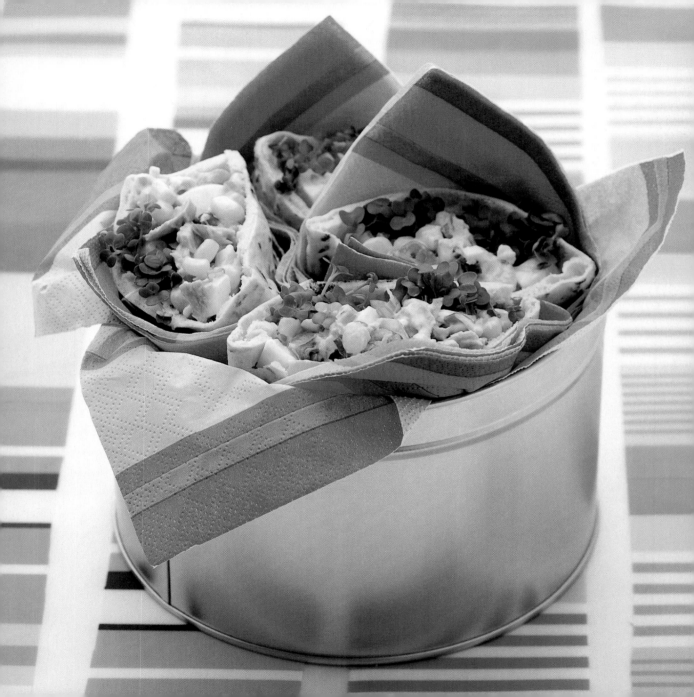

# pita pockets stuffed with tuna, egg, and corn

Pita pockets with a nutritious filling make a good snack or light lunch. This tuna mix is delicious.

◯ **Makes 4 pita pockets**

*2 eggs*
*one 6-ounce can tuna in oil, drained*
*½ cup corn*
*2 tablespoons mayonnaise*
*1 teaspoon white wine vinegar*
*4 scallions, chopped*
*salt and freshly ground black pepper*
*few drops of Tabasco sauce*
*alfalfa sprouts (optional)*
*2 pita breads*

Put the eggs in a saucepan of cold water and bring to a boil. Reduce the heat and simmer for 7 to 8 minutes. Drain and cool under cold water. Peel the eggs when cold.

Meanwhile, flake the tuna with a fork and mix with the corn, mayonnaise, white wine vinegar, scallions, salt and pepper, and Tabasco sauce. Roughly chop the hard-boiled eggs and add to the tuna mix with the sprouts (if using), stirring well.

Cut the pita breads in half to make four pita pockets and divide the mixture among them.

**LUNCH BOX LOWDOWN**
Add a personal touch to your child's lunch. Tuck in a note, stickers, or joke or send a special treat labeled "Share with a friend." Pack fun napkins, decorate lunch bags with stickers, or draw a face on a banana with a marker pen.

# wraps

**Wraps make a great alternative to sandwiches, and you can find soft flour tortillas in the bread section of most supermarkets. Other good tortilla fillings are:**

• Tuna with corn, cucumber, and mayonnaise

• Chicken, avocado, lettuce, and mayonnaise with toasted pine nuts

## quick turkey wraps

▽ **Makes 2 wraps**
*2 small flour tortillas*
*1 tablespoon mayonnaise*
*2 thin slices deli roast turkey*
*handful of shredded lettuce*
*2 heaping tablespoons grated Cheddar cheese*

Lay out the tortillas and spread them with the mayonnaise. Lay a turkey slice on top of each tortilla and cover with some lettuce and grated cheese. Roll up and wrap in foil or plastic wrap.

---

**LUNCH BOX LOWDOWN**

It's a good idea to wrap one end of the tortilla in foil so that the filling doesn't fall out when it's eaten. Your child can unfold the foil as he eats the wrap.

---

## chicken tortillas

▽ **Makes 2 wraps**
*1½ teaspoons olive oil (plus extra to drizzle)*
*1 small red onion, thinly sliced*
*1 small clove garlic, crushed*
*1 small skinless, boneless chicken breast,*
*    cut into strips*
*1 teaspoon balsamic vinegar*
*pinch of dried oregano*
*salt and freshly ground black pepper*
*6 cherry tomatoes, cut into quarters*
*4 sun-dried tomatoes in oil, drained and chopped*
*3 basil leaves, torn into pieces*
*2 small flour tortillas*
*mayonnaise*
*a little shredded iceberg lettuce*

Heat the oil in a small frying pan and sauté the red onion for 2 minutes. Add the garlic and chicken and sauté for 3 to 4 minutes or until the chicken is cooked through. Add the balsamic vinegar and oregano and season to taste.

Meanwhile, mix together the cherry tomatoes, sun-dried tomatoes, and basil, drizzle some olive oil on top, and add a pinch of black pepper.

Spread the tortillas with a little mayonnaise. Divide the chicken and tomato mixture between the two tortillas and top with some lettuce. Roll up the tortillas and wrap tightly in foil or plastic wrap.

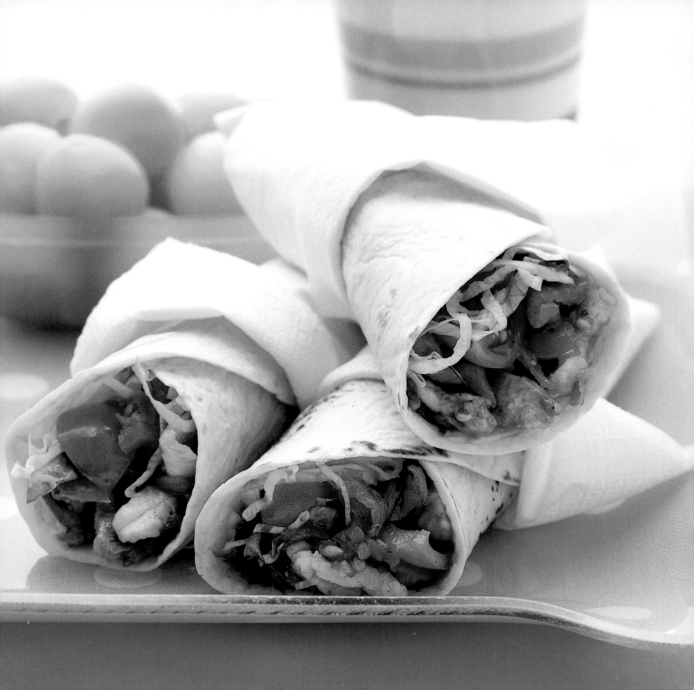

## oriental turkey wraps

This is a simple recipe using leftover turkey. Turkey meat keeps best if stripped off the bone. When cold, if wrapped in waxed paper and foil, it should keep in the fridge for up to four days. Dark turkey meat contains twice as much iron and zinc as white. Plum sauce comes in jars and is available at most supermarkets.

◯ **Makes 4 wraps**
*8 ounces shredded dark turkey meat*
*some plum sauce*
*few drops of sesame oil*
*¼ cup mayonnaise*
*1½ teaspoons soy sauce*
*½ small cucumber, peeled and cut into matchsticks*
*2 large scallions, finely sliced*
*1½ teaspoons toasted sesame seeds (optional)*
*4 small flour tortillas*

Arrange the turkey on a baking sheet. Spread a little plum sauce on top and sprinkle with sesame oil, then broil for about 5 minutes until browned.

Mix together the mayonnaise and soy sauce. Stir in the turkey, cucumber, and scallions and sprinkle the sesame seeds (if using) on top.

Heat the tortillas for a few seconds in a microwave or dry frying pan. Arrange the filling down one side of each tortilla and roll up. Cut in half diagonally and wrap in foil.

## shrimp and avocado wrap

◯ **Makes 1 wrap**
*¼ avocado, chopped*
*1 teaspoon lemon juice*
*½ medium tomato, seeded and diced*
*1 teaspoon sliced scallion*
*¼ cup small peeled cooked shrimp*
*1 tablespoon mayonnaise*
*½ teaspoon ketchup*
*salt and freshly ground black pepper*
*1 small flour tortilla*

Put the avocado and lemon juice into a small bowl. Toss together until the avocado is coated with the lemon juice. Add the tomato, scallion, shrimp, mayonnaise, and ketchup and combine. Season with salt and pepper.

Spoon the mixture onto the tortilla and roll up. Cut in half and wrap in foil. Advise your child to unwrap the tortilla slowly as he eats, to keep the filling contained.

### LUNCH BOX LOWDOWN
Some 45 percent of school pupils say they prefer a packed lunch to a school meal. If your child is a fussy eater, it can be much better to give him a packed lunch containing the food he likes rather than letting him go hungry because he doesn't like school lunches.

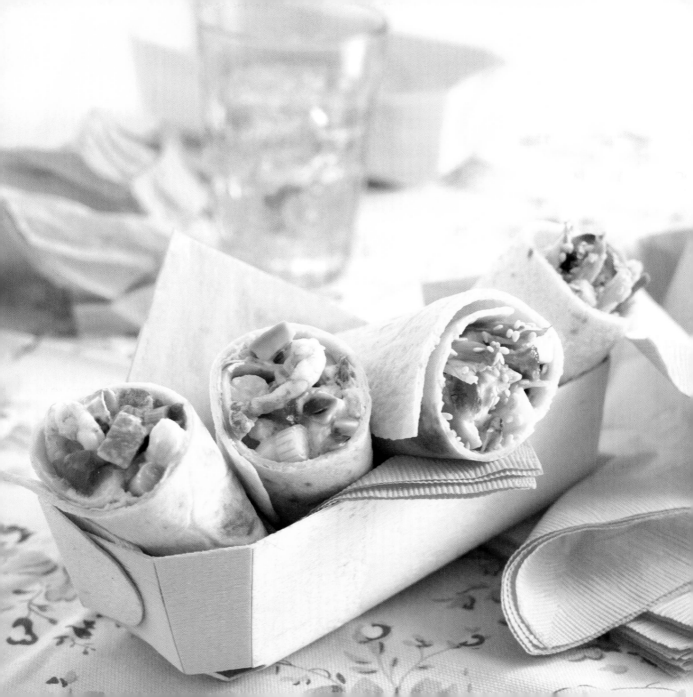

# southwestern chicken wraps

◯ **Makes 2 wraps**
*1 small skinless, boneless chicken breast*
*1 teaspoon McCormick Fajita Seasoning*
*2 teaspoons olive oil*
*½ teaspoon lemon or lime juice*
*2 tablespoons sour cream*
*2 teaspoons mayonnaise*
*½ teaspoon lime juice*
*salt and freshly ground black pepper*
*2 small flour tortillas*
*handful of shredded romaine or iceberg lettuce*
*1 medium tomato, seeded and sliced into strips*

Place the chicken breast between two layers of plastic wrap and flatten with a rolling pin to ¼ inch thick. Mix together the fajita seasoning, oil, and lemon or lime juice and rub over the chicken. Leave to stand for 10 minutes.

Preheat the broiler to high and broil the chicken, 5 inches from the heat source, for 5 to 6 minutes on each side until cooked through. Allow to cool, then refrigerate until needed (can be made up to two days in advance).

Slice the cold chicken into thin strips. Mix together the sour cream, mayonnaise, and lime juice and season with salt and pepper. Spread on top of the tortillas, then scatter the lettuce and tomato on top. Lay the chicken strips down the center and roll up. Wrap in foil or plastic wrap.

# chicken wrap with tomato pesto

You could use red pesto or sun-dried-tomato paste in this wrap, and instead of diced fresh tomato, you could add two chopped sun-dried tomatoes.

◯ **Makes 1 wrap**
*1 to 1½ tablespoons mayonnaise*
*½ teaspoon red pesto or sun-dried-tomato paste*
*small squeeze of lemon juice*
*¼ cup shredded cooked chicken*
*½ tomato, diced*
*1 small flour tortilla*
*some shredded iceberg lettuce*

Mix together the mayonnaise, pesto, and lemon juice. Stir in the cooked chicken and diced tomato. Heat the tortilla for 20 seconds in a microwave or about 15 seconds on each side in a dry frying pan.

Arrange the chicken down one side of the tortilla, cover with shredded lettuce, and roll up. Cut the tortilla in half diagonally. Wrap in foil or plastic wrap.

> **LUNCH BOX LOWDOWN**
> Wraps make a nice change from ordinary sandwiches, and if you put the fillings into separate bowls, children will have fun making them up themselves.

## chicken caesar wrap

This wrap uses the classic Caesar dressing with chicken. As a shortcut, you could use a store-bought Caesar salad dressing to mix with the chicken.

◯ **Makes 1 wrap**
1½ tablespoons mayonnaise
1 teaspoon water
small squeeze of lemon juice
few drops of Worcestershire sauce (optional)
1½ teaspoons freshly grated Parmesan cheese
1 small flour tortilla
¼ cup shredded cooked chicken
2 tablespoons grated carrot
some shredded iceberg lettuce

Make the dressing by mixing together the mayonnaise, water, lemon juice, Worcestershire sauce (if using), and Parmesan. Heat the tortilla for 20 seconds in a microwave or about 15 seconds on each side in a dry frying pan.

Mix together the chicken and carrot and toss with the dressing. Arrange the chicken along one side of the tortilla. Top with the shredded lettuce and roll up. Wrap in foil or plastic wrap.

## cream cheese, banana, and honey wrap

This is also very tasty if, instead of honey, you use 1 teaspoon of dulce de leche—a delicious caramel spread that you can buy in jars or cans in most supermarkets.

◯ **Makes 1 wrap**
1 small flour tortilla
2 tablespoons cream cheese
½ teaspoon honey
1 small banana, sliced

Warm the tortilla for 20 seconds in a microwave or about 15 seconds on each side in a dry frying pan. Mix together the cream cheese and honey and spread over half the tortilla. It will melt slightly, as the tortilla is warm. Arrange the sliced banana on top and roll up. Wrap in foil or plastic wrap.

> **TOP SNACKING TIPS**
> Keep healthy snacks like vegetable sticks and hummus dip, or a tasty pasta salad, in the fridge where your children can help themselves.

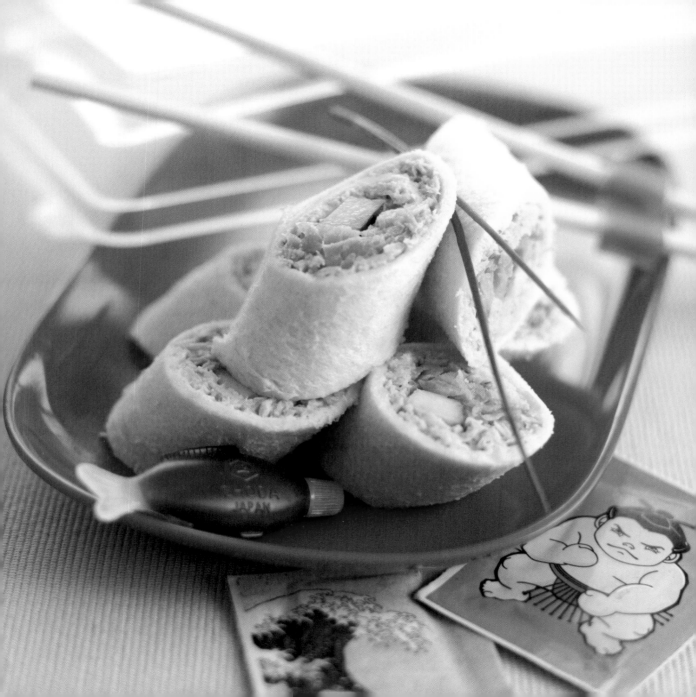

# kiddie sushi-style rolls

⬭ **Makes 1 portion**

*2 slices white bread, crusts removed*
*half a 6-ounce can tuna in oil, drained*
*2 tablespoons mayonnaise*
*1½ tablespoons ketchup*
*2 drops Tabasco sauce (or to taste)*
*2-inch piece of cucumber, cut into strips*
*2-inch piece of carrot, peeled and coarsely grated*

Using a rolling pin, flatten the bread until it is about ¼ inch thick.

Mix the tuna together with 1 tablespoon of the mayonnaise, the ketchup, and the Tabasco. Spread the remaining 1 tablespoon mayonnaise over the bread and then spoon the tuna in a line about ½ inch from one edge of each slice. Arrange the cucumber strips on one side of the tuna and the grated carrot on the other side. Roll up from the filled end and press down to seal. Trim the ends to neaten using a sharp knife, then cut into three little rolls.

You can prepare this the night before, wrap the rolls in plastic wrap, then cut each one into three pieces in the morning.

### Other good fillings to try are:

- Canned salmon mixed with a little mayonnaise, ketchup, and chopped scallion with cucumber strips

- Strips of Cheddar cheese with slices of tomato and cucumber

- Hummus with grated carrot, shredded lettuce, and chopped tomato

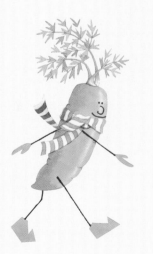

**LUNCH BOX LOWDOWN**
Avoid giving your child too many processed foods, as they tend to contain few nutrients, too much salt, sugar, and saturated fat, and a lot of additives.

# egg heads

**This is a fun way to prepare egg sandwiches. Get your children to help you design the faces.**

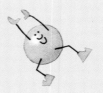

## How do you tell if an egg is fresh?

Place an egg in a bowl or pan with enough cold water to cover the egg.

- If the egg lies on its side on the bottom, it's very fresh.
- If the egg stands up and bobs on the bottom, it isn't quite as fresh.
- If the egg floats on the surface, it should be thrown away.

◯ **Makes 4 egg heads**
*7 eggs*
*¼ cup mayonnaise*
*salt and freshly ground black pepper*
*4 slices bread, buttered*

### Some ideas for face decorations
*sliced bell pepper*
*grated carrot*
*olives*
*salami*
*gherkins*
*chives*
*basil*
*peas*
*celery*

Put the eggs in a saucepan of cold water and bring to a boil. Reduce the heat and simmer for 7 to 8 minutes. Place the eggs in a bowl under cold running water until cool. Peel off the shells.

Slice two of the eggs using an egg slicer or a knife. Set aside eight of the slices to make the eyes. Place the remaining pieces in a bowl with the remaining five eggs. Mash with a fork and add the mayonnaise. Season with salt and pepper to taste.

Cover all four slices of bread with egg mayonnaise. Make the faces using the toppings shown in the photo for inspiration!

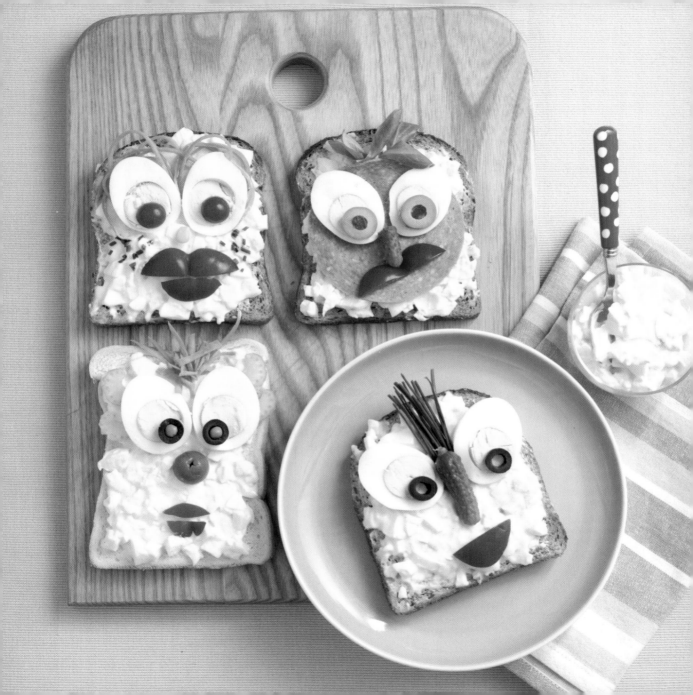

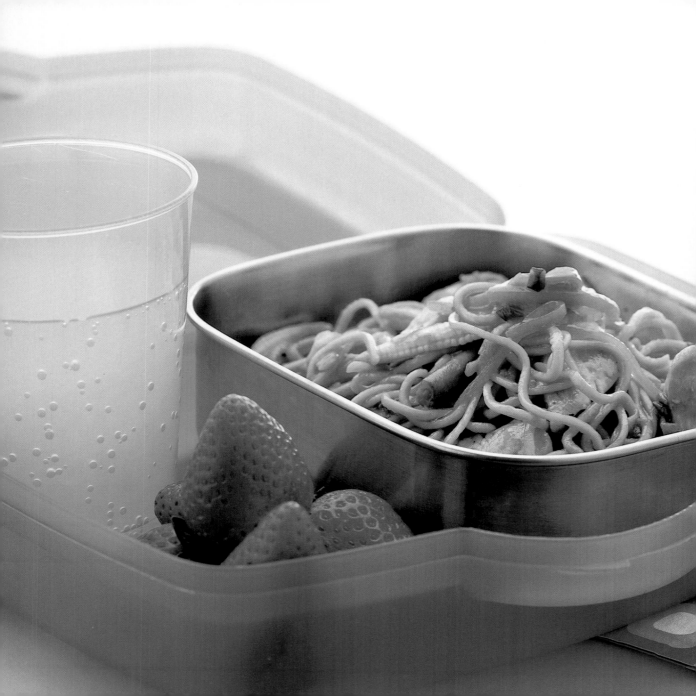

# savory specialties

If you pack a thermos in the lunch box, you can give your child something hot, like soup or pasta, on a cold winter's day.

*sweet-and-sour chicken noodles (see page 42)*

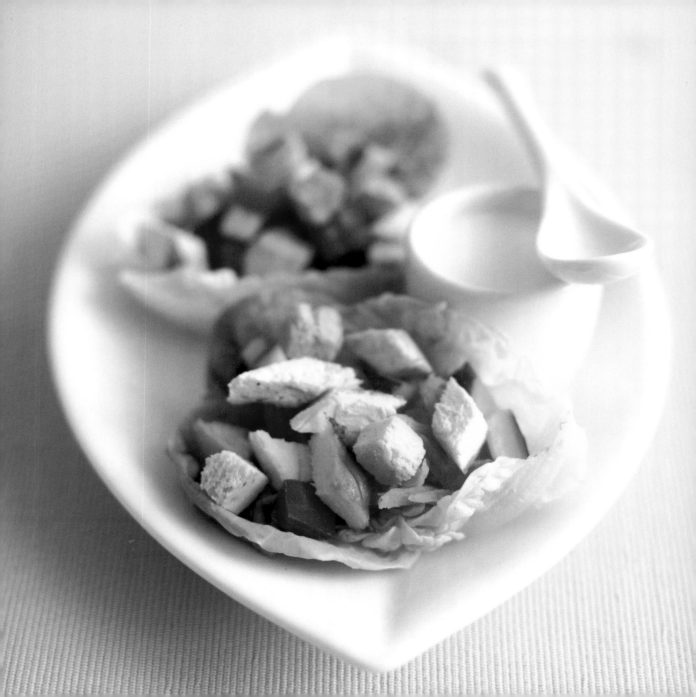

# caesar salad lettuce cups

⬭ **Makes 2 portions**

*1 small skinless, boneless chicken breast*

### Marinade

*1 tablespoon olive oil*
*1 teaspoon lemon juice*
*salt and freshly ground black pepper*

### Caesar dressing

*3 tablespoons mayonnaise*
*1 teaspoon lemon juice*
*2 teaspoons water*
*2 teaspoons freshly grated Parmesan cheese*
   *(plus extra to serve)*
*2 or 3 drops Worcestershire sauce (to taste)*
*salt and freshly ground black pepper*

### Extras you can add

*grated carrot, diced cucumber, diced apple,*
*chopped cherry tomatoes, sliced scallion*

*2 Boston lettuce leaves*
*croutons*

Place the chicken breast between two layers of plastic wrap and flatten with a rolling pin to ¼ inch thick. Mix together the marinade ingredients, add the chicken, and marinate for 30 minutes. Heat a griddle and brush with oil. Remove the chicken from the marinade and cook for 3 to 4 minutes on each side or until cooked through. Whisk the dressing ingredients in a bowl. Dice the chicken and toss it in the dressing. Add extras if you wish. Spoon onto the lettuce leaves, add a few croutons, and sprinkle with Parmesan.

# salsa chicken lettuce cups

⬭ **Makes 6 portions**

*1 cooked chicken breast*
*6 small Boston lettuce leaves*
*2½ tablespoons tomato salsa*
*1 heaping tablespoon sour cream*

Cut the chicken into bite-size pieces. Fill the lettuce leaves with the chicken and top with the salsa and sour cream.

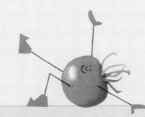

### LUNCH BOX LOWDOWN

Children tend to consume too much salt in their diet. High levels of salt can make them vulnerable to health problems such as high blood pressure, heart disease, and strokes later in life. Many of the foods manufactured specifically for packed lunches—like cheese spreads, processed ham, and salt-and-vinegar chips—are very high in salt. Check labels and avoid foods that have a high salt content. Recommended salt intake is about ½ teaspoon, or 3 g (1.2 g sodium), per day for 4- to 6-year-olds, or about 1 teaspoon, or 5 g (2 g sodium), for 7- to 10-year-olds. Eating foods that contain potassium helps to balance the effect of salt in the body. Bananas and dried apricots are good sources of potassium.

# sweet-and-sour chicken noodles

○ **Makes 2 portions**

*Sauce*

*1 teaspoon red wine vinegar*
*1 tablespoon soy sauce*
*1 tablespoon ketchup*
*2 tablespoons pineapple juice*
*1/2 teaspoon superfine sugar*
*1 teaspoon cornstarch*

*1 tablespoon vegetable oil*
*1 small skinless, boneless chicken breast,*
*    cut into strips*
*salt and freshly ground black pepper*
*2 tablespoons finely sliced scallion*
*1/4 red bell pepper, cut into matchsticks*
*1 carrot, peeled and cut into matchsticks*
*1/4 cup green beans, topped, tailed, and halved*
*2 ounces Chinese bean thread noodles*

Mix together all the sauce ingredients and set aside. Heat half the oil in a wok or frying pan, lightly season the chicken, and sauté for 3 to 4 minutes until cooked. Remove from the pan.

Add the remaining oil and stir-fry the vegetables for 3 minutes. Pour the sauce in, bring to a boil, then reduce the heat and simmer for 1 minute.

Cook the noodles according to the package directions, drain, and mix together with the chicken and vegetables.

*(see photograph on pages 38–39)*

# chicken chunks on a stick

You can make these for dinner and wrap a couple in foil for your child's lunch box the next day. You might prefer to remove the food from the skewer before packing it—not as much fun to eat, but better than an accident with the stick. This tasty marinated chicken is also good in a wrap with some mayonnaise, shredded lettuce, and tomato.

○ **Makes 4 sticks**

*2 tablespoons soy sauce*
*1 heaping tablespoon dark brown sugar*
*1 tablespoon lime or lemon juice*
*1 1/2 teaspoons vegetable oil*
*1 small clove garlic, crushed*
*2 small skinless, boneless chicken breasts,*
*    cut into chunks*

Put the soy sauce and sugar into a small saucepan and heat gently, stirring until the sugar has dissolved. Remove from the heat and stir in the lime or lemon juice, vegetable oil, and garlic. Marinate the chicken for at least 1 hour or overnight.

Soak four bamboo skewers in water. Thread the chunks of chicken onto the skewers, place on a broiler pan, brush with the marinade, and broil for 4 to 5 minutes on each side, basting with marinade halfway through, until the chicken is thoroughly cooked. Alternatively, you can cook the marinated chicken breasts whole on a griddle, but flatten them before marinating.

# hidden-vegetable tomato sauce

⬭ **Makes 5 portions**
❄ **Sauce suitable for freezing**

*1 tablespoon olive oil*
*½ red onion, chopped*
*2 carrots, peeled and grated*
*½ small red bell pepper, cored, seeded, and chopped*
*1 small zucchini, chopped*
*1 cup canned crushed tomatoes*
*¼ cup vegetable broth*
*1 teaspoon sugar*
*1 teaspoon balsamic vinegar*
*1 teaspoon dried oregano*
*¼ cup mascarpone cheese*

*12 ounces pasta (½ cup per portion)*

This delicious tomato sauce flavored with mascarpone cheese is a great way to get children to eat vegetables, because the sauce makes the vegetables invisible and what children can't see, they can't pick out. You can leave out the mascarpone if you prefer.

### LUNCH BOX LOWDOWN

You can control what goes into your child's lunch box, but you can't control what goes into your child. I know it may seem obvious, but make sure that you send your child to school with food that she likes. It's often a good idea, time permitting, to let your child help to pack her own lunch box or perhaps discuss with her the night before what she would like to include.

Heat the oil in a saucepan and sauté the onion for about 4 minutes. Add the carrots and bell pepper and cook for 3 minutes. Add the zucchini, tomatoes, broth, and sugar and simmer, covered, for 20 minutes. Add the balsamic vinegar and oregano and continue to cook for 5 minutes.

Transfer the sauce to a food processor and blend until smooth. Return to the saucepan, add the mascarpone cheese, and heat gently, stirring continuously, until the cheese has melted into the sauce. Divide the sauce into five portions. Cook ½ cup pasta according to the package directions, toss with sauce, and transfer to a thermos. (Freeze the remaining sauce until needed.)

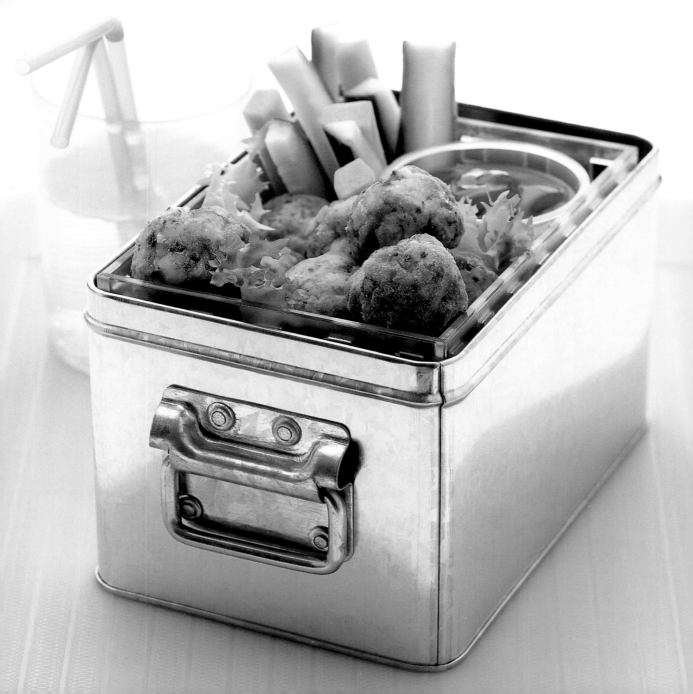

# finger-picking chicken balls

The grated apple adds a delicious flavor to these chicken balls and they are very popular eaten hot or cold. Include a little ketchup in a separate plastic container for dipping.

▽ **Makes about 20 chicken balls**
❋ **Suitable for freezing**
*1 large Granny Smith apple, peeled and grated*
*2 small skinless, boneless chicken breasts,*
    *cut into chunks*
*1 onion, finely chopped*
*1 tablespoon chopped fresh parsley*
*1 teaspoon fresh or ¹/₂ teaspoon dried thyme*
    *(optional)*
*¹/₂ cup fresh white bread crumbs*
*1 chicken bouillon cube dissolved in 1 tablespoon*
    *boiling water*
*salt and freshly ground black pepper*
*flour for coating*
*vegetable oil for frying*

Using your hands, squeeze out some of the excess liquid from the grated apple. Mix the apple with the chicken, onion, parsley, thyme (if using), bread crumbs, and chicken bouillon and roughly chop in a food processor for a few seconds. Season with a little salt and pepper.

With your hands, form the mixture into about 20 balls, roll in flour, and fry in shallow oil for about 10 minutes, until lightly golden and cooked through.

# chicken quesadillas

▽ **Makes 2 quesadillas**
*1¹/₂ teaspoons sunflower oil*
*1 small skinless, boneless chicken breast,*
    *cut into small strips*
*¹/₂ onion, sliced*
*¹/₄ red bell pepper, thinly sliced*
*1 tablespoon balsamic vinegar*
*¹/₂ teaspoon light brown sugar*
*2 tablespoons tomato salsa*
*2 small flour tortillas*
*¹/₂ cup grated Cheddar cheese*

Heat the oil in a wok or large frying pan and stir-fry the chicken for 2 minutes. Add the onion and cook for 2 minutes more. Add the bell pepper and cook for another 2 to 3 minutes. Add the balsamic vinegar and brown sugar and cook for 1 minute.

Spread 1 tablespoon of the salsa over half of each tortilla and sprinkle ¹/₄ cup of the cheese on top. Divide the chicken mixture between the two tortillas and sprinkle with the remaining ¹/₄ cup cheese. Roll up.

Broil for 1¹/₂ to 2 minutes on each side to warm the tortilla and melt the cheese.

> **LUNCH BOX LOWDOWN**
> Studies show that children who drink lots of water are better at concentrating and remembering. Give your child a bottle of water to take into an exam, and avoid foods that dehydrate, such as potato chips.

# sticky drumsticks

This tasty marinade gives drumsticks a delicious flavor. They can be marinated and cooked the day before and refrigerated. Halve the quantity of marinade for two drumsticks. Wrap them in foil or plastic wrap.

▽ **Makes 4 drumsticks**

*Marinade*
*3 tablespoons plum jam*
*1 tablespoon soy sauce*
*1 teaspoon lemon juice*
*few drops of Tabasco sauce*
*1 tablespoon sesame seeds*

*4 chicken drumsticks, skinned*

Mix together all the ingredients for the marinade in a bowl.

Wash the chicken drumsticks and pat them dry with paper towels. Score each one several times using a sharp knife and mix into the marinade. Leave for 1 to 2 hours or overnight in the fridge.

Turn on the broiler to high. Place the marinated chicken on a baking sheet 4 to 5 inches below the heating element. Broil the chicken for about 20 minutes, basting with the marinade halfway through and turning occasionally to prevent burning.

# chicken drumsticks with barbecue sauce

▽ **Makes 6 drumsticks**
*6 chicken drumsticks*

*Marinade*
*3 tablespoons ketchup*
*1 tablespoon sunflower oil*
*1 tablespoon rice wine vinegar*
*1 tablespoon soy sauce*
*2 tablespoons honey*
*1 teaspoon paprika*
*1 clove garlic, crushed*

Wash the chicken drumsticks, pat them dry with paper towels, and score each one three times using a sharp knife.

Thoroughly mix together all the ingredients for the marinade. Coat the drumsticks in the marinade and leave for 30 minutes or overnight in the fridge.

Preheat the oven to 400°F.

Line a baking sheet or roasting pan with foil. Place the drumsticks and marinade in the pan. Bake for 35 to 40 minutes, basting occasionally with the marinade, until the chicken is thoroughly cooked.

> **LUNCH BOX LOWDOWN**
> Put extra foil around the ends of chicken drumsticks so that your child can hold them without getting sticky fingers.

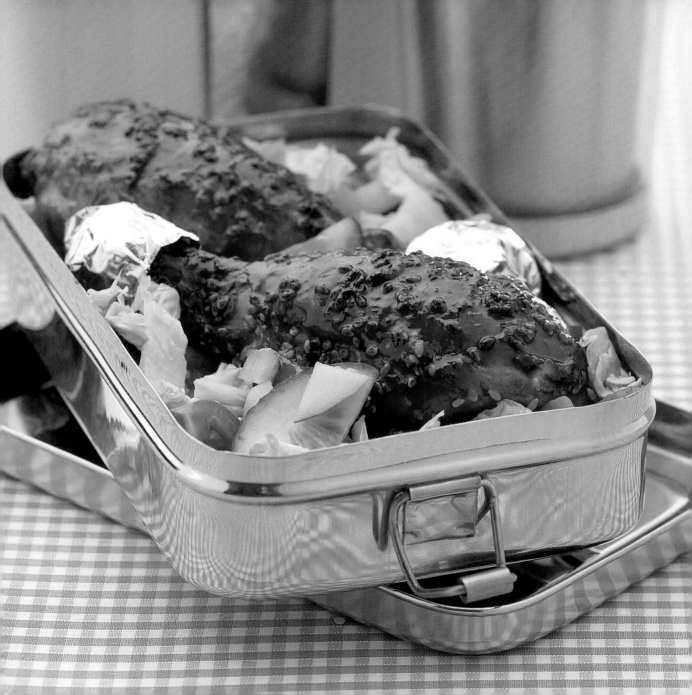

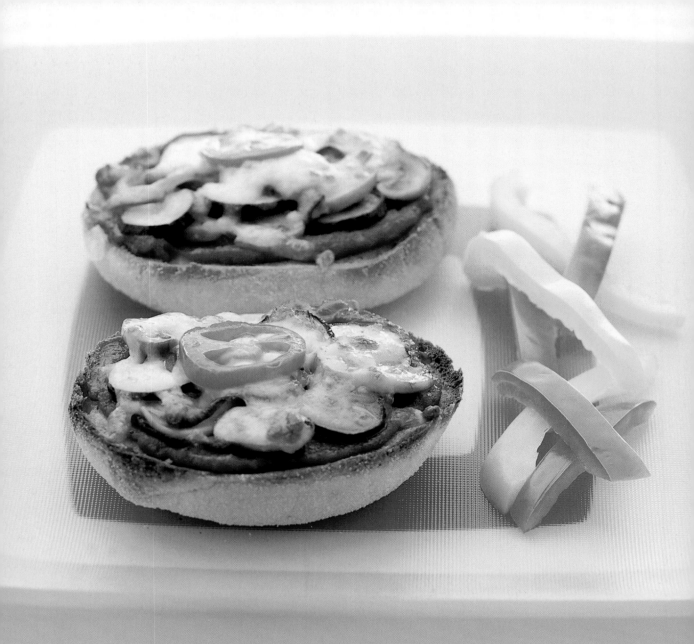

# mini muffin pizzas

You can use whatever toppings your child likes for these mini pizzas. Try ham and pineapple, tuna and corn, or cherry tomato and pepperoni. You can also make simple pizzas by spreading the muffins with ketchup, arranging sliced cherry tomatoes on top, covering with grated Cheddar cheese, and cooking under a broiler until lightly golden.

▽ **Makes 2 mini pizzas**
*1 English muffin, cut in half*
*1 tablespoon tomato paste*
*1 teaspoon red pesto*
*1 tablespoon olive oil*
*½ small red onion, sliced*
*2 to 3 button mushrooms, sliced*
*½ small zucchini, thinly sliced*
*salt and freshly ground black pepper*
*1 slice ham or salami, cut into pieces (optional)*
*½ cup ready-grated mozzarella or*
*    grated Cheddar cheese*

Toast the muffin until golden and leave to cool. Preheat the broiler. Mix the tomato paste and red pesto and spread over the muffin halves. Heat the olive oil in a frying pan and cook the onion, mushrooms, and zucchini until softened and golden.

Add the seasonings and then divide the vegetables between the muffin halves and scatter the ham or salami and mozzarella or Cheddar over the top. Place under the broiler and cook for 4 minutes or until golden and bubbling.

# 15-minute pizzas

Split and toasted English muffins make a good base for these individual pizzas. You can vary the toppings, maybe adding extras such as sliced mushrooms, strips of ham, or pepperoni.

▽ **Makes 8 mini pizzas**
*4 English muffins*
*¼ cup pizza sauce*
*2 scallions, finely sliced*
*¼ cup canned corn*
*8 cherry tomatoes, sliced*
*salt and freshly ground black pepper*
*¾ cup ready-grated Cheddar and mozzarella,*
*    mixed, or grated Cheddar cheese*
*olive oil to drizzle*
*4 sprigs of fresh basil (optional)*

Preheat the oven to 350°F.

Cut the muffins in half, arrange on a baking sheet, and spread with the pizza sauce. Sprinkle the scallions, corn, and cherry tomatoes on top, season with a little salt and pepper, and top with the cheese. Drizzle over a little olive oil. Bake for about 10 minutes. Decorate with the basil if you like.

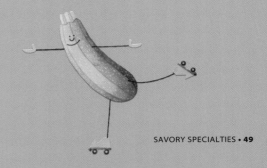

# cheesy muffins

As a variation on these savory muffins, try making cheese and corn muffins: Add 2 tablespoons maple syrup to the milk mixture, increase the cheese quantity to 1 cup, use 5 scallions, and stir in ¾ cup canned corn.

▽ **Makes 10 muffins**
*¼ cup milk*
*¼ cup vegetable oil*
*½ cup plain yogurt*
*2 eggs*
*1¼ cups all-purpose flour*
*½ teaspoon baking soda*
*1½ teaspoons baking powder*
*¼ teaspoon paprika*
*½ teaspoon salt*
*Freshly ground black pepper*
*1 cup grated Cheddar cheese*
*4 scallions, sliced*
*⅓ cup grated Parmesan cheese*

Preheat the oven to 350°F. Line a muffin pan with paper cups.

Combine the milk, oil, yogurt, and eggs in a bowl. In another bowl, sift together the flour, baking soda, baking powder, paprika, and salt and pepper. Stir in the Cheddar cheese and scallions.

Add the liquid ingredients to the flour mixture and mix quickly before spooning into the paper cups. Sprinkle the Parmesan on top and bake for 20 minutes.

# tuna melt

This recipe is quick, easy, and nutritious and my children love it. You could use Greek-style yogurt instead of crème fraîche if you wish.

▽ **Makes 4 melts**
*one 6-ounce can tuna in water*
*2 tablespoons ketchup*
*2 tablespoons crème fraîche*
*1 or 2 scallions, finely sliced*
*2 English muffins*
*¼ cup grated Cheddar cheese*

Drain the tuna and flake into small pieces. Mix together with the ketchup, crème fraîche, and scallions.

Cut the muffins in half and toast them. Spread with the tuna mixture and sprinkle the grated cheese on top. Place the muffins under the broiler and heat until the cheese is golden and bubbling.

> ## TOP SNACKING TIP
> If your child is always famished after school and can't wait to get home and have something to eat, pack an after-school snack in the lunch box. Choose something that won't spoil, like a peanut butter sandwich, muffin, or cereal bar, or fruit.

# muffins with creamy scrambled eggs

Instead of using English muffins, you could use split bagels.

▽ **Makes 2 muffins**
*2 English muffins*
*4 eggs*
*3 tablespoons heavy cream*
*a little salt and freshly ground black pepper*
*a little butter or margarine*

***Optional extras***
*snipped fresh chives*
*thin strips of smoked salmon*
*chopped tomato*
*strips of ham*

Cut the muffins in half and toast them. Meanwhile, break the eggs into a small bowl, add the cream, and season with salt and pepper. Whisk lightly. Melt some butter in a heavy-bottomed, nonstick saucepan over medium heat. Pour in the egg mixture, leave for a few seconds, and then stir briskly with a wooden spoon until softly set. At this stage, you could stir in one of the optional extras.

Spread the muffins with a little butter and pile the scrambled eggs on top.

# toasted ham and cheese muffins

Instead of sprinkling the ham with Worcestershire sauce, you can spread the muffin halves thinly with mustard, then top with ham and cheese and broil until golden.

▽ **Makes 1 muffin**
*1 English muffin*
*a little butter or margarine*
*2 thin slices ham*
*few drops of Worcestershire sauce*
*3 tablespoons grated Cheddar cheese*

Turn on the broiler. Cut the muffin in half, arrange the halves upside down on a broiler pan, and heat for 1 minute. Remove them from the heat, turn over, and spread with a little butter or margarine. Divide the ham between the muffin halves and add a few drops of Worcestershire sauce. Top with the grated cheese and broil for 3 to 4 minutes until golden.

> **LUNCH BOX LOWDOWN**
> If your children take a packed lunch to school every day, by the time they are sixteen, you will have prepared more than 2,500 lunch boxes.

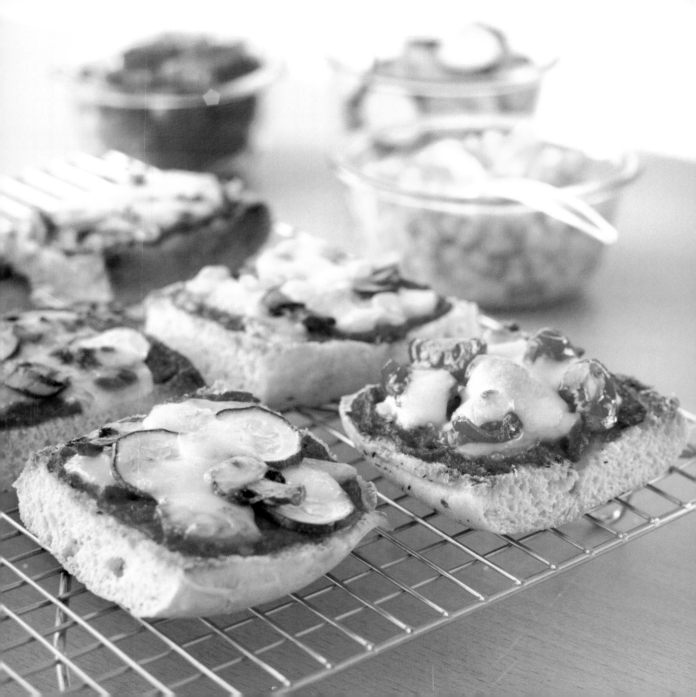

# individual focaccia pizzas

Split toasted focaccia bread makes a good pizza base. You could also use split toasted English muffins. You can top the pizza with a hidden-vegetable tomato sauce (choose between the one given here and the one on page 43), then let your child choose her favorite toppings—cherry tomatoes, corn, mushrooms, zucchini, and ham all work well. If you don't have time to make the sauce, simply use a good-quality pizza sauce. I prefer to cover the pizza with firm mozzarella, rather than the soft balls, as it has more flavor.

◯ **Makes about 8 mini pizzas**

*Hidden-vegetable tomato sauce*
1 tablespoon olive oil
1 small onion, finely chopped
1 clove garlic, crushed
¼ cup diced red bell pepper
¼ cup diced zucchini
one 14.5-ounce can diced tomatoes
1 tablespoon sun-dried-tomato paste or tomato sauce
2 large pinches dried thyme
1 teaspoon sugar
a little salt and freshly ground black pepper

*focaccia bread cut into about 8 squares*
1¼ cups ready-grated mozzarella (firm variety)
      or grated Cheddar cheese

In a large saucepan, heat the olive oil, add the onion, and sauté for 5 minutes. Add the garlic, bell pepper, and zucchini and cook for a further 5 minutes. Add the diced tomatoes, tomato paste, thyme, and sugar, and simmer for 25 to 30 minutes until the sauce is very thick. Remove from the heat, blitz with a hand blender, and season to taste with a little salt and pepper.

Place the focaccia bread under the broiler, cut side facing up, and lightly toast. Spread each slice with 1 tablespoon of the sauce. Cover with any toppings of your child's choice and the mozzarella or Cheddar and broil for 1 to 2 minutes until golden.

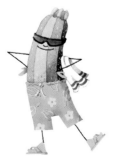

# chicken satay

🥣 **Makes 8 skewers**

*Marinade*
1 tablespoon soy sauce
1 clove garlic, crushed
1 1/2 tablespoons lemon juice
1 tablespoon peanut butter
1 tablespoon honey

2 skinless, boneless chicken breasts

*Peanut sauce*
1 tablespoon vegetable oil
1/2 onion, finely chopped
1/2 teaspoon crushed dried red pepper
1/4 cup water
1/4 cup coconut milk
1/2 cup crunchy or smooth peanut butter
1 teaspoon light brown sugar

**Chicken doesn't have to be covered in bread crumbs or batter to appeal to children. They love chicken skewers. Try them with this delicious marinade and dipping sauce.**

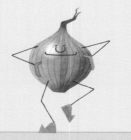

**LUNCH BOX LOWDOWN**
Pasta salads, sandwich fillings, and fruit compotes can be prepared the night before to save time in the morning. You could even include some leftovers from the evening meal, such as soup in a thermos, chicken skewers, or a Spanish omelet.

Mix together all the ingredients for the marinade. To flatten the chicken breasts, place them between two layers of plastic wrap and carefully bash with a rolling pin. Cut each one lengthwise into four or five strips. Marinate the chicken for 15 to 30 minutes. Soak eight bamboo or wooden skewers in cold water for about 20 minutes—this stops them from becoming burnt or charred during cooking.

To make the peanut sauce, heat the vegetable oil in a pan and sauté the onion and red pepper for 4 minutes. Add the remaining ingredients. Bring to a boil, stirring, then simmer for 2 minutes or until thickened.

Turn on the broiler. Thread the chicken strips onto the skewers and broil for about 8 minutes, turning occasionally. Serve the skewers with the dipping sauce and rice.

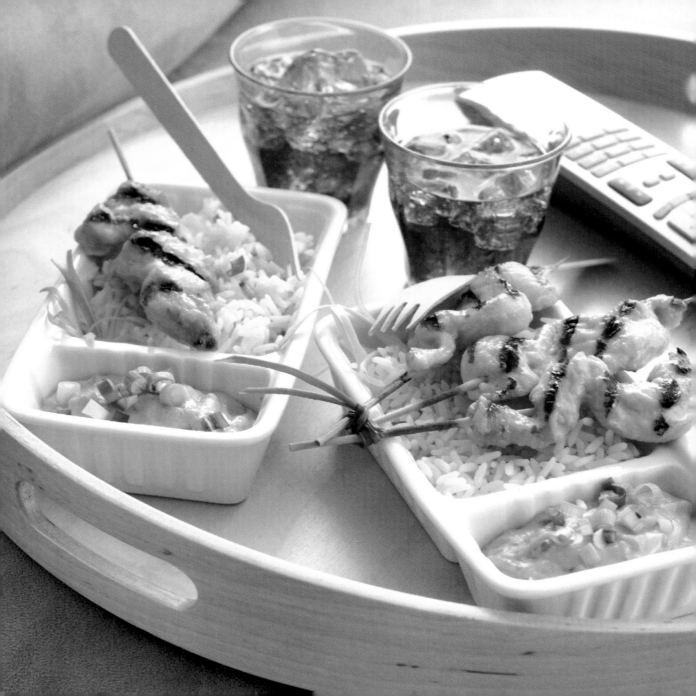

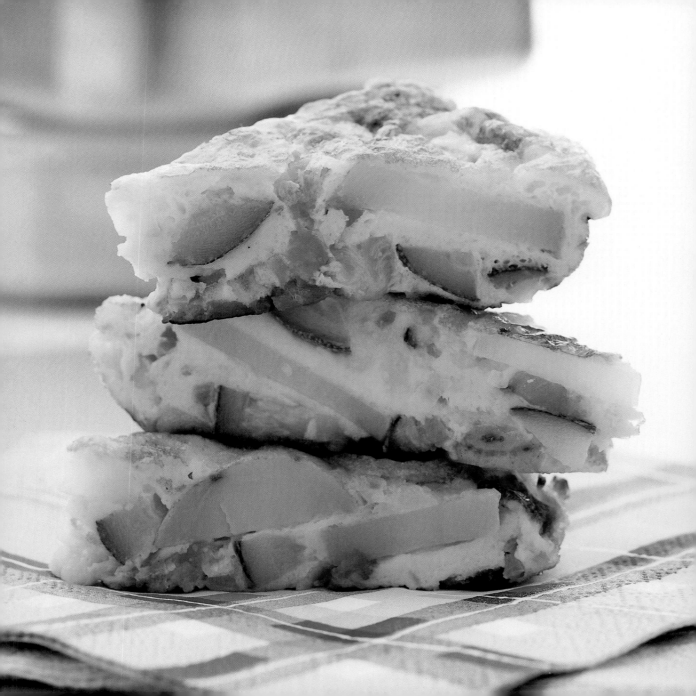

# spanish omelet with potatoes, zucchini, and tomato

◯ **Makes 6 portions**

*4 to 6 baby Yukon Gold potatoes*
*1 tablespoon olive oil*
*1 small onion, finely chopped*
*1 zucchini, diced or grated*
*2 tomatoes, peeled, seeded, and roughly chopped*
*4 eggs*
*1 tablespoon milk*
*2 tablespoons grated Parmesan cheese*
*salt and freshly ground black pepper*

Bring a saucepan of lightly salted water to a boil, add the potatoes, reduce the water to a simmer, and cook the potatoes for about 12 minutes until tender. Drain, allow to cool, and then slice.

Heat the oil in an ovenproof nonstick medium frying pan. Add the onion and sauté for 2 minutes. Then add the zucchini and sauté for another 6 minutes (4 minutes if using grated zucchini). When the zucchini is cooked, add the tomatoes and cook for 2 minutes, then stir in the sliced potatoes.

Beat the eggs together with the milk, Parmesan, and a little seasoning. Pour the egg mixture over the vegetables and cook over medium heat for about 4 minutes until the underside of the eggs has set. Meanwhile, preheat the broiler to high. Place the frying pan under the broiler with the oven door open and the handle sticking out and cook for about 3 minutes until golden and set. Slide the omelet out onto a plate. When the omelet is cold, cut into wedges and wrap in foil.

**Spanish omelets are good eaten hot or cold. You could cook this for supper and then wrap a piece up in foil and store in the fridge ready for your child's lunch box the next day. Try this with other vegetables, too, such as diced bell pepper, peas, and diced potato.**

## LUNCH BOX LOWDOWN

Girls begin their growth spurt between the ages of 8 and 10, in contrast to boys, who start theirs a little later, around the age of 12 years. Peak bone growth occurs around the age of 12 in girls and 14 in boys. So, it is very important that children between 7 and 12 years old get enough calcium in their diet—the equivalent of 3¾ cups of milk a day. One 6-ounce container of yogurt and 2 slices of hard cheese provide the same amount of calcium as 2 cups of milk.

# mummy's ramen noodles

Always popular with kids, but the ones you buy are really high in salt. It takes only a few minutes to make your own, and it's fun to serve in cups.

◯ **Makes 2 portions**
*6 ounces fine Chinese-style dried egg noodles or*
  *straight-to-the-wok fine thread noodles*
*1 cup chicken broth*
*1 tablespoon dark soy sauce*
*⅓ cup frozen peas*
*½ cup canned or frozen corn*
*⅔ cup shredded cooked chicken*
*1 scallion, thinly sliced (optional)*
*1 teaspoon cornstarch*

Cook the noodles according to the package directions (or use precooked noodles). Drain and set aside. Put the broth, soy sauce, peas, corn, and chicken in a saucepan over medium heat. Stir in the scallion (if using). Bring to a simmer and cook for 2 minutes.

In a small bowl, mix the cornstarch with 2 teaspoons cold water and add to the contents of the pan. Cook, stirring, for 1 minute or until the liquid thickens slightly. Add the noodles and reheat briefly, stirring. Transfer to a bowl to serve, or use individual plastic cups.

# mini quiches

These mini quiches freeze well and are the perfect size for lunch boxes. You could use diced ham or tomato instead of corn.

◯ **Makes 6 mini quiches**
❄ **Suitable for freezing**
*one 15-ounce package refrigerated piecrust*
*3 tablespoons canned corn*
*½ cup grated sharp Cheddar cheese*
*2 tablespoons finely sliced scallion*
*½ cup milk*
*1 large egg, plus 1 egg yolk*
*salt and freshly ground black pepper*

Preheat the oven to 350°F. Using a 3½-inch round cookie cutter, cut out six circles from the piecrust. Press them into six greased cups of a muffin pan.

Divide the corn among the piecrust cups. Sprinkle the Cheddar on top, then the scallion. Put the milk into a bowl, add the eggs, and beat until thoroughly combined. Season well with salt and pepper to taste. Carefully pour the egg mixture into the piecrust cups, making sure not to overfill.

Bake the quiches for 20 to 25 minutes until slightly puffed and the piecrust is golden around the edges. Run a knife around the edge of each cup to loosen, then leave for 10 minutes before removing from the pan and placing on a wire rack to cool. As soon as they are cold, transfer to the fridge.

If necessary, freeze in an airtight container for up to one month and thaw overnight in the fridge.

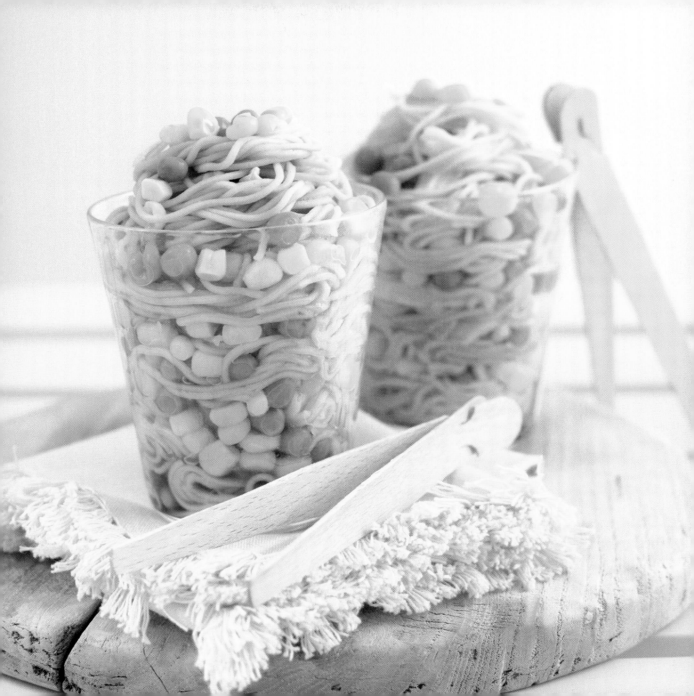

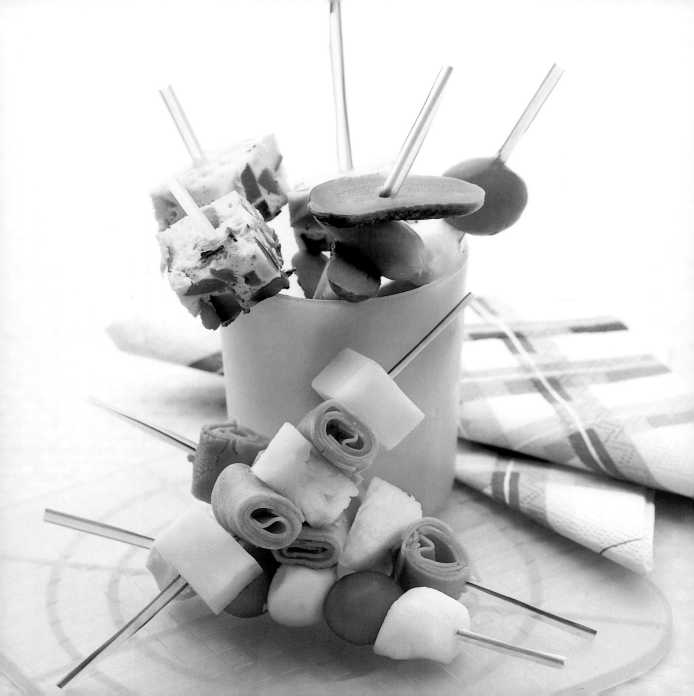

# luscious lunch on a stick

You can make up "kebabs" with many different foods, using straws instead of skewers. They are quick to put together and easy to pack in the lunch box. Add a container of ketchup or a dip for extra flavor. Here are some ideas for you to try, but feel free to make up your own combinations, choosing healthy foods that your child enjoys. There is plenty of scope for your children to help with this task.

- *Slices of ham or turkey rolled up and interspersed with cubes of cheese and wedges of pineapple (optional)*
- *Cherry tomatoes and chunks of cucumber and mozzarella cheese*
- *Slices of cooked sausage and gherkin*
- *Pieces of carrot, celery, cucumber, bell pepper, and baby corn*
- *Squares of Spanish omelet (see page 57)*
- *Salami, cubes of mozzarella cheese, and cherry tomatoes*

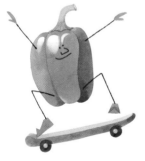

# honey and soy toasted seeds

These flavored seeds are very nutritious and taste wonderful. Sunflower seeds are a good source of the antioxidant vitamin E, which boosts the immune system and is vital for healthy brain function. Pumpkin seeds contain omega-3 fatty acids, which are crucial for brain development. The seeds will keep for two weeks in an airtight container.

▽ **Makes 4 portions**
*1 tablespoon sunflower oil*
*½ cup sunflower seeds*
*½ cup pumpkin seeds*
*1 tablespoon honey*
*1 tablespoon soy sauce*

Heat the oil in a nonstick frying pan, add the seeds, and cook, stirring continuously, for about 2 minutes until the seeds are lightly browned. Remove from the heat, add the honey and soy sauce, and return to the heat for 1 minute. Spread out on a baking sheet and leave to cool. This prevents the seeds from sticking together. Store in an airtight container.

> **LUNCH BOX LOWDOWN**
> To add some excitement to lunchtime, pack little surprises in your child's lunch box from time to time: stickers; a novelty pen, eraser, or sharpener; a mini notebook; or a joke. Simple gestures like this will let your child know that your thoughts are with her, even when she is at school.

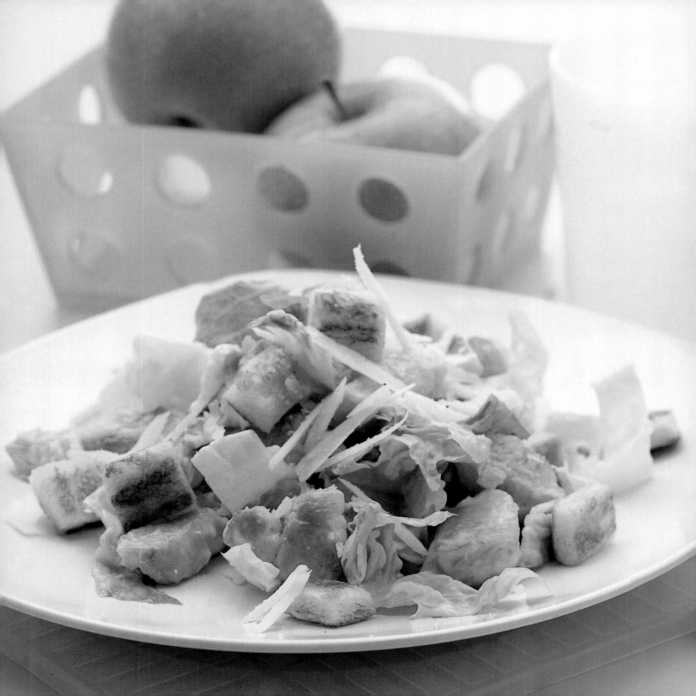

# crunchy salads

Instead of sandwiches, try making tasty pasta, rice, or couscous salads for your child's lunch box. The secret of getting him to enjoy eating salad is to find an irresistible salad dressing—there are some fabulous dressings in this chapter.

*chicken caesar salad (see page 66)*

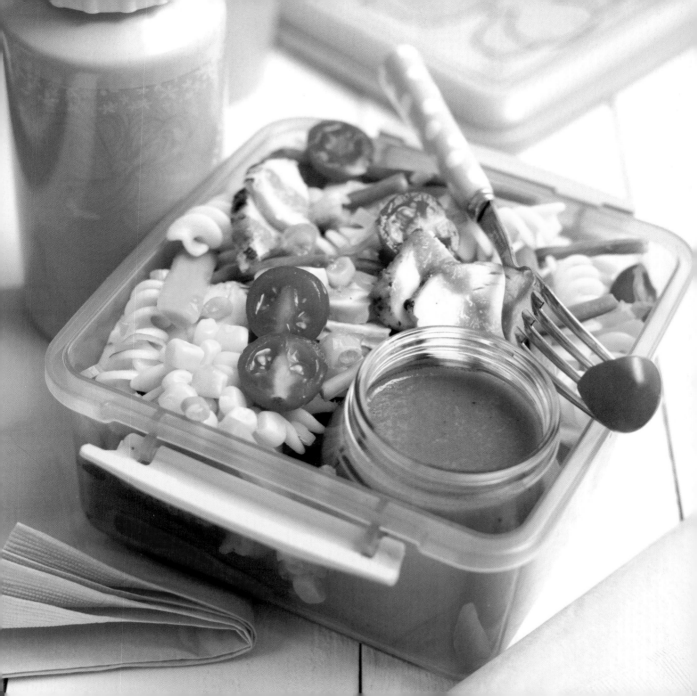

# pasta salad with annabel's dressing

This salad dressing is pure magic and I can't make enough of it to please my children. They love it—not only as a salad dressing, but also on rice, chicken, and pasta and as a dip with raw vegetables like sticks of cucumber, carrot, and bell pepper. I usually make up a large batch of the dressing and keep it in a bottle in the fridge.

**Dressing**
½ small onion, finely chopped
¼ cup vegetable oil
1½ tablespoons rice wine vinegar
1 tablespoon soy sauce
1 tablespoon chopped celery
scant teaspoon finely chopped fresh gingerroot
1 tablespoon water
1½ teaspoons tomato paste
1½ teaspoons superfine sugar
1½ teaspoons lemon juice
salt and freshly ground black pepper

5 ounces pasta shapes
½ cup canned or frozen corn
1 carrot, peeled and cut into thin strips
½ cup topped and tailed green beans
6 small cherry tomatoes, halved
1 small skinless, boneless chicken breast, cooked and diced

First make the dressing. Combine all the dressing ingredients in a food processor and blend until smooth.

Bring a saucepan of lightly salted water to a boil and cook the pasta according to the package directions. If you are using frozen corn, cook it in a saucepan of boiling water or in the microwave.

Put the carrot and green beans in a steamer (two-tiered if possible) for about 5 minutes until just cooked. Drain the pasta and mix it together with the carrot, beans, tomatoes, corn, and chicken. Toss with ½ cup of the salad dressing.

# chicken caesar salad

The croutons and dressing for this salad can be made the evening before. All you need to do in the morning is mix all the ingredients together and toss with the dressing. You could even use ready-made croutons, in which case all you need to do is assemble the ingredients—so simple!

▽ **Makes 1 portion**
1 tablespoon olive oil
1 slice thick white bread (crusts trimmed), chopped into small cubes

*Dressing*
2 tablespoons mayonnaise
1 tablespoon grated Parmesan cheese
1 teaspoon lemon juice
$\frac{1}{2}$ small clove garlic, crushed
$\frac{1}{8}$ teaspoon Dijon mustard
few drops of Worcestershire sauce
few drops of Tabasco sauce

$\frac{1}{2}$ cup diced cooked chicken
$\frac{1}{2}$ head romaine lettuce, sliced or torn into pieces
1 tablespoon grated Parmesan cheese

Heat the olive oil in a small nonstick frying pan and add the cubes of bread. Fry, turning occasionally, until golden brown. Remove with a slotted spoon and drain on paper towels.

In a bowl, combine all the dressing ingredients. Mix together the chicken and lettuce and toss with most of the dressing. Pack the grated Parmesan and the croutons in a separate plastic container for your child to scatter over the salad at lunchtime.

(see photograph on pages 62–63)

**LUNCH BOX LOWDOWN**
Pack the dressing separately from the salad and let your child mix the two himself just before he starts to eat. This way, the salad will remain crisp.

# pasta shell salad with chicken and corn

⌒ **Makes 4 portions**

*1 small skinless, boneless chicken breast*
*1 cup chicken broth*
*5 ounces tiny shell pasta*
*½ cup topped and tailed green beans*
*½ cup canned corn*
*3 scallions, finely chopped (optional)*

*Dressing*
*¼ cup light olive oil*
*1 tablespoon balsamic vinegar*
*1 tablespoon soy sauce*
*½ teaspoon superfine sugar*
*a little salt and freshly ground black pepper*

Poach the chicken in the chicken broth for 7 to 8 minutes until cooked through. Remove the chicken with a slotted spoon and allow to cool a little. Shred the chicken.

Cook the pasta according to the package directions. Steam the green beans for about 5 minutes until just cooked. Drain the pasta and mix together with the chicken, green beans, corn, and scallions (if using).

Whisk together all the dressing ingredients and toss with the pasta salad.

Corn is a useful source of several of the B vitamins, especially folate. It also provides significant levels of fiber, vitamin C, and potassium. This salad is ideal for keeping in the fridge so that your children can help themselves when they feel hungry. To save time, use ready-cooked chicken. You may use turkey instead, if you wish.

**LUNCH BOX LOWDOWN**

If your child likes to share his food or trade with friends, include an extra "valuable" treat such as Rice Krispies squares, chocolate muffins, or popcorn. Why not label it "For a Friend"?

# turkey pasta salad with honey and soy dressing

▽ **Makes 4 portions**

*8 ounces fusilli pasta*
*1 bunch broccoli, cut into small florets*

*Honey and soy dressing*
*5 tablespoons olive oil*
*2 tablespoons soy sauce*
*1¹/₂ tablespoons honey*
*1¹/₂ tablespoons lemon juice*
*a little freshly ground black pepper*

*³/₄ cup halved cherry tomatoes*
*1 cup canned corn*
*4 ounces cooked turkey, chopped into small pieces*
*3 scallions, finely sliced*

Cook the pasta according to the package directions. Steam the broccoli for 3 to 4 minutes or blanch in lightly salted water for a couple of minutes. Meanwhile, whisk together all the dressing ingredients.

Drain the pasta, place in a large bowl, and combine with the broccoli, cherry tomatoes, corn, turkey, and scallions. Toss with the dressing and serve.

**If you make this dressing for supper, it will still be fresh the following day, so you can put a small container in your child's lunch box. You will find moist slices of cooked turkey at any supermarket delicatessen counter.**

> **LUNCH BOX LOWDOWN**
> Some schools operate a healthy-eating policy with regard to packed lunches. For example, they might ban potato chips or chocolate. It might be an idea to discuss this policy with some of the other parents and suggest a trial at your child's school.

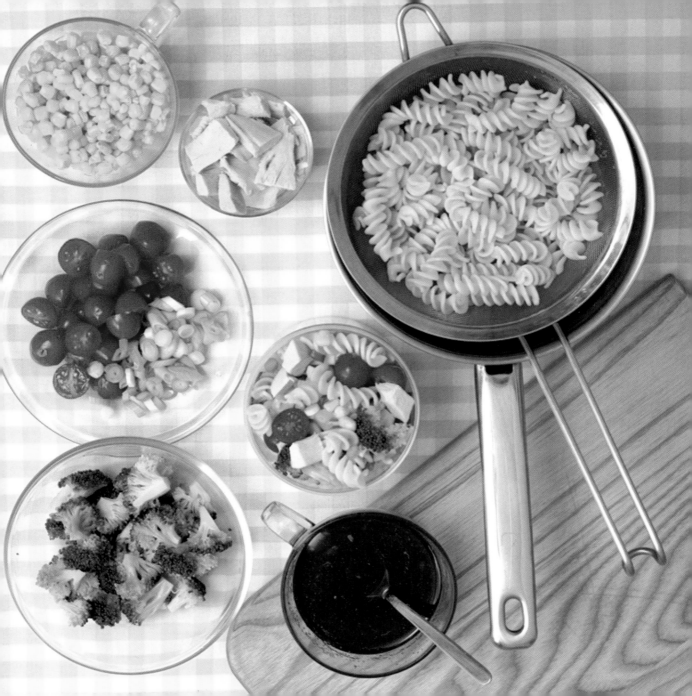

# tuna pasta salad

⬭ **Makes 1 portion**

*1 cup fusilli pasta*
*1 cup halved cherry tomatoes*
*2 scallions, sliced*
*⅓ cup canned corn*
*one 6-ounce can tuna, drained and flaked*
*small handful of torn fresh basil leaves*

**Thousand Island dressing**
*½ cup mayonnaise*
*2 tablespoons sour cream*
*1 heaping tablespoon ketchup*
*¼ teaspoon lemon juice*
*2 or 3 drops Tabasco sauce (to taste)*
*¼ small red bell pepper, finely diced*
*½ large scallion, finely diced*
*salt and freshly ground black pepper*

Cook the pasta according to the package directions. Drain and mix with the cherry tomatoes, scallions, corn, tuna, and basil.

Mix together all the dressing ingredients. You will find that you have more dressing than you need— the remainder will keep well in the fridge. Toss the pasta salad with the dressing.

# carrot and cucumber salad

The Japanese make this salad using seaweed and cucumber. However, seaweed is pretty hard to find, so I have used carrot instead. You could also use bean sprouts or shredded Chinese cabbage.

If using, toast the sesame seeds in a dry frying pan, stirring occasionally, for a few minutes until golden.

⬭ **Makes 2 portions**

*1 large carrot, peeled*
*½ English or hothouse seedless cucumber*

**Dressing**
*1 tablespoon toasted sesame seeds (optional)*
*1 tablespoon soy sauce*
*1 tablespoon rice wine vinegar*
*1 tablespoon sunflower oil*
*1 tablespoon honey*
*1 teaspoon mirin*
*1 teaspoon sesame oil*

Using a swivel vegetable peeler, make thin strips of carrot and cucumber. Mix together the dressing ingredients and toss with the salad.

# pasta with shrimp and avocado

A shrimp cocktail with a difference. If your child doesn't like avocado, leave it out and use chopped tomatoes or cherry tomatoes instead.

⬭ **Makes 3 portions**

*7 ounces pasta shapes*
*1 ripe avocado, chopped into ¹/₂-inch cubes*
*1¹/₂ cups small peeled cooked shrimp*
*1 head Boston lettuce, cut into ¹/₂-inch pieces*
*1 tablespoon snipped fresh chives*

*Sauce*
*2 tablespoons ketchup*
*1 teaspoon soy sauce*
*few drops of Tabasco sauce*
*¹/₂ teaspoon Worcestershire sauce*
*¹/₃ cup heavy cream*
*¹/₄ cup mayonnaise*
*squeeze of lemon juice, to taste*

*paprika to garnish*

Cook the pasta according to the package directions. Mix together the avocado, shrimp, lettuce, and chives.

Mix together all the sauce ingredients. Toss with the salad and sprinkle a little paprika on top.

---

**LUNCH BOX LOWDOWN**

Children sometimes like to eat breakfast for lunch—try packing some of your child's favorite cereal and a small carton of milk.

This is the most delicious, easy-to-prepare chicken salad. It's great for lunch or supper and is perfect for transporting in a child's lunch box. Pasta provides a good source of energy, and if you add chicken or tuna, you have a good mix of complex carbohydrate and protein.

**LUNCH BOX LOWDOWN**

Instead of putting a package of potato chips or some chocolate cookies in your child's lunch box, try offering popcorn, rice cakes, yogurt-covered raisins, or dried apricots.

# chicken salad with corn, pasta, and cherry tomatoes

◯ **Makes 6 portions**

*2 small skinless, boneless chicken breasts*
*2¹/₂ cups chicken broth*

**Dressing**
*3 tablespoons olive oil*
*1 tablespoon white wine vinegar*
*¹/₂ teaspoon Dijon mustard (optional)*
*¹/₂ teaspoon sugar*
*salt and freshly ground black pepper*
*1 tablespoon chicken broth from the poaching liquid*

*1 cup pasta bows, cooked and cooled*
*1 cup canned or cooked frozen corn*
*18 small cherry tomatoes, halved*
*2 scallions, finely sliced*
*¹/₂ head Boston lettuce, shredded*

Poach the chicken in the broth for about 10 minutes, then allow to cool completely. Remove the chicken with a slotted spoon and cut into bite-size pieces (this can be prepared the night before).

To make the dressing, whisk together all the ingredients. Combine the remaining salad ingredients with the chicken and toss with the dressing.

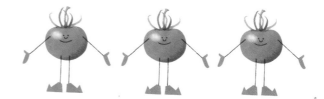

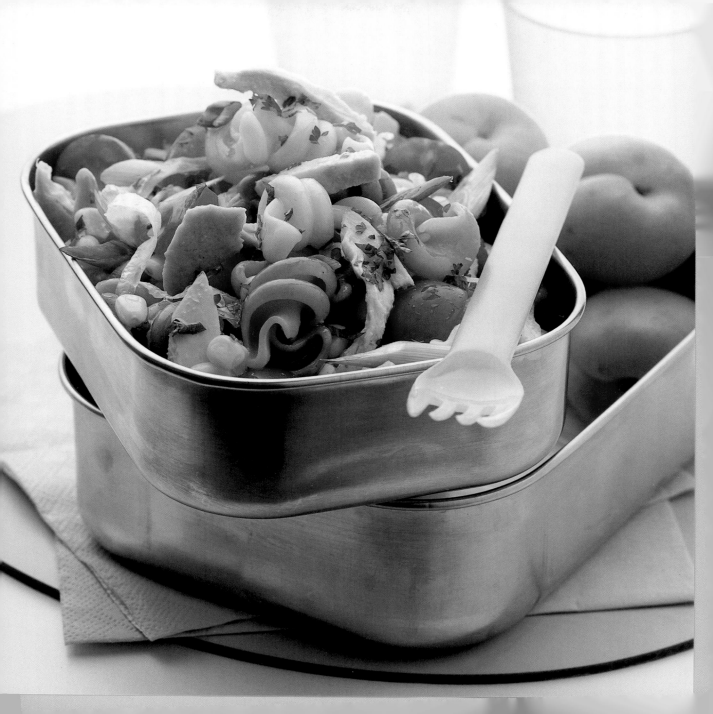

# confetti couscous salad

◯ **Makes 2 portions**

*¼ cup couscous*
*½ cup hot vegetable broth*
*2 tablespoons diced red bell pepper*
*½ medium carrot, peeled and diced*
*2 scallions, sliced*
*1 tablespoon raisins*
*1½ tablespoons pine nuts, toasted*

**Dressing**
*1 tablespoon olive oil*
*1½ teaspoons lemon juice*
*½ teaspoon honey*
*salt and freshly ground black pepper*

Put the couscous into a bowl. Pour the broth over it and leave to stand for about 5 minutes or according to the package directions.

Fluff up the couscous with a fork. Stir in the bell pepper, carrot, scallions, raisins, and pine nuts.

Whisk together the dressing ingredients and stir into the couscous. Season to taste.

**LUNCH BOX LOWDOWN**

According to a recent survey on lunch boxes, just over 25 percent of lunch boxes contain no fruit or vegetables. Very few parents pack only healthy foods. However, the majority (65 percent) attempt to balance, giving children items such as potato chips or chocolates but also giving fruit or vegetables. Almost three in ten mothers are "sweet avoiders," allowing chips and other savory snacks, but not cookies or chocolates.

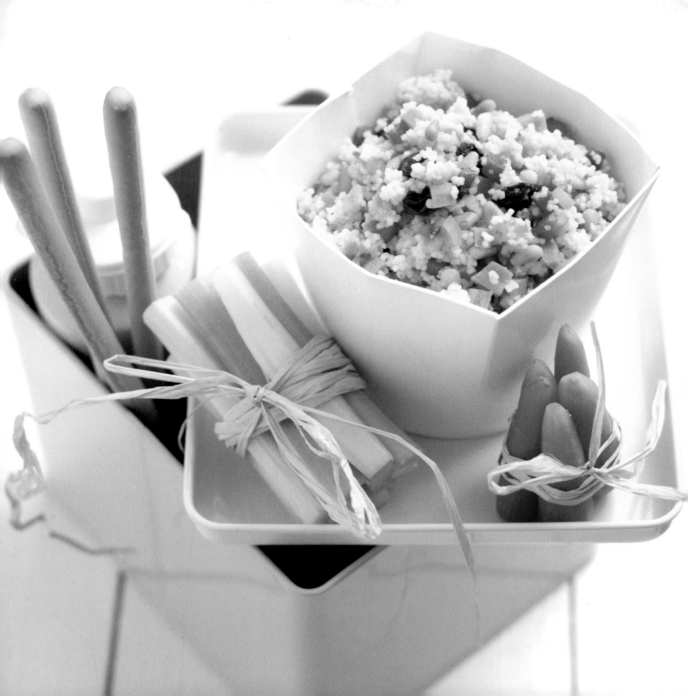

# chef's salad with turkey and cheese

You can add other ingredients to this salad if you like:

- Try some cooked corn or cherry tomatoes.
- Include a boiled egg instead of the cheese.
- Replace the turkey with chopped slices of ham.

As an alternative dressing, mix some mayonnaise with a little white wine vinegar or use the dressing from the recipe for pasta with shrimp and avocado (see page 71).

▽ **Makes 1 portion**
*Dressing*
*1 teaspoon red wine vinegar*
*1 1/2 teaspoons honey*
*2 tablespoons olive oil*
*1 teaspoon orange juice*
*salt and freshly ground black pepper*

*1/4 cup cubed cooked turkey*
*4 cherry tomatoes, halved*
*1 1/2-inch piece of English or hothouse seedless cucumber, cubed*
*1/2 head Boston lettuce, chopped*
*1/4 cup cubed Edam cheese*
*1 scallion, finely sliced*
*handful of alfalfa sprouts*

To make the dressing, whisk together all the ingredients.

Mix together all the salad ingredients and toss in as much of the dressing as you like (there will probably be some dressing left over).

---

**LUNCH BOX LOWDOWN**
Turn leftovers like plain cooked pasta or couscous into a salad by adding vegetables such as steamed broccoli, corn, and cherry tomatoes, and, for protein, some chicken or ham. Then just toss in your favorite dressing.

# crunchy salad

As a child, I used to love this salad. If you are short of time, you don't need to blanch the cabbage. If you wish, you could leave out the cabbage and simply mix grated carrot and raisins with the dressing.

▽ **Makes 1 portion**
*½ cup shredded white cabbage*

**Dressing**
*2 tablespoons mayonnaise*
*1½ teaspoons vegetable oil*
*1 teaspoon lemon juice*

*1 carrot, peeled and grated*
*1½ tablespoons raisins*

Blanch the cabbage in boiling water for 1 to 2 minutes and then drain. Using a fork, whisk together the dressing ingredients. Combine the cabbage, carrot, and raisins and toss with the dressing.

# mixed salad

My children love this salad dressing, which is flavored with soy sauce. If you like, you can add other ingredients to the salad, such as chopped chicken or turkey, avocado, toasted pine nuts, and sunflower seeds.

▽ **Makes 1 portion**
*¼ cup topped and tailed green beans*
*¼ cup chopped iceberg lettuce*
*¼ cup canned or cooked frozen corn*
*4 cherry tomatoes, halved*
*1 small carrot, peeled and grated*
*1 hard-boiled egg, quartered*

**Dressing**
*2 tablespoons olive oil*
*1½ teaspoons soy sauce*
*1½ teaspoons balsamic vinegar*
*pinch of superfine sugar*
*freshly ground black pepper*

Steam the green beans for about 4 minutes until tender. Mix together with the lettuce, corn, tomatoes, carrot, and egg.

Whisk together the dressing ingredients and toss with the salad.

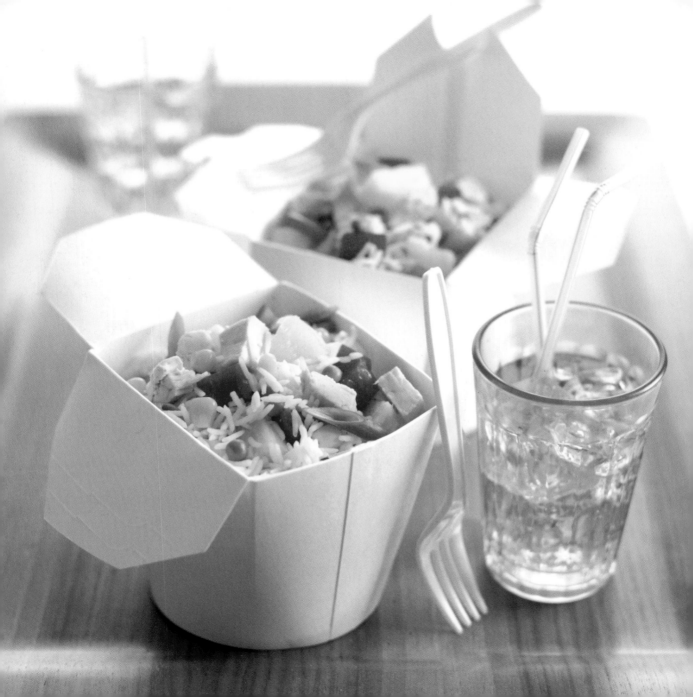

# chicken and rice salad

◯ **Makes 2 to 3 portions**

½ cup long-grain white rice
3 large scallions, sliced
¼ cup diced cooked chicken
¼ cup cooked frozen peas
¼ cup canned corn
¼ cup pineapple chunks in juice, drained
    (reserve the juice)
1 tomato, seeded and diced

**Dressing**
2 tablespoons sunflower or canola oil
2 tablespoons pineapple juice (from the can)
1 teaspoon lemon juice
salt and freshly ground black pepper

Cook the rice according to the package directions and leave to cool. Mix together with the rest of the ingredients for the chicken salad. Whisk together the dressing ingredients and toss with the salad.

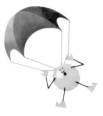

# rice salad with corn, raisins, and cashew nuts

◯ **Makes 1 to 2 portions**

½ cup basmati rice
4 scallions, sliced
¾ cup canned corn
½ cup cashew nuts, roughly chopped
2 tablespoons raisins

**Dressing**
2 tablespoons olive oil
1 tablespoon plus 1 teaspoon lemon juice
1 teaspoon snipped fresh chives
salt and freshly ground black pepper

Cook the rice according to the package directions. Rinse well in cold water and leave to drain thoroughly. Transfer to a bowl.

Stir in the scallions, corn, cashew nuts, and raisins. Whisk together the dressing ingredients and stir into the rice salad. Season to taste.

**LUNCH BOX LOWDOWN**
If your child wears braces, avoid putting hard, crunchy food such as a whole apple in his lunch box.

# spinach salad with mango and strawberries

◯ **Makes 2 to 3 portions**

*2 tablespoons pine nuts*
*2 cups baby spinach or mixed salad greens*
*2 tablespoons diced red onion*
*1 small or ½ large ripe mango, peeled and chopped*
*5 strawberries, hulled and sliced*
*2 tablespoons dried cranberries*

*Dressing*
*3 tablespoons vegetable oil*
*1 tablespoon balsamic vinegar*
*1 teaspoon sugar*
*salt and freshly ground black pepper*

Heat a dry frying pan and toast the pine nuts, stirring continuously, for about 2 minutes until lightly browned.

Meanwhile, in a bowl, combine the spinach, red onion, mango, strawberries, and cranberries. To make the dressing, whisk together the oil, balsamic vinegar, sugar, and seasonings. Then toss the salad with the dressing and sprinkle the pine nuts over the top.

This salad has some lovely flavors and is easy to prepare. Mangoes are very rich in antioxidants; an average-size fruit provides the minimum adult daily requirement of vitamin C, two-thirds of the vitamin A, and nearly half the vitamin E. Vitamin C boosts iron absorption, which can aid concentration. Vitamin A helps to boost the immune system, fight infections, and promote good eyesight, and vitamin E promotes normal cell growth and development. Ripe mango is easy to digest and is also a good source of fiber.

**LUNCH BOX LOWDOWN**
When children are dehydrated, their concentration levels drop. Give your child a brightly colored water bottle to take to school.

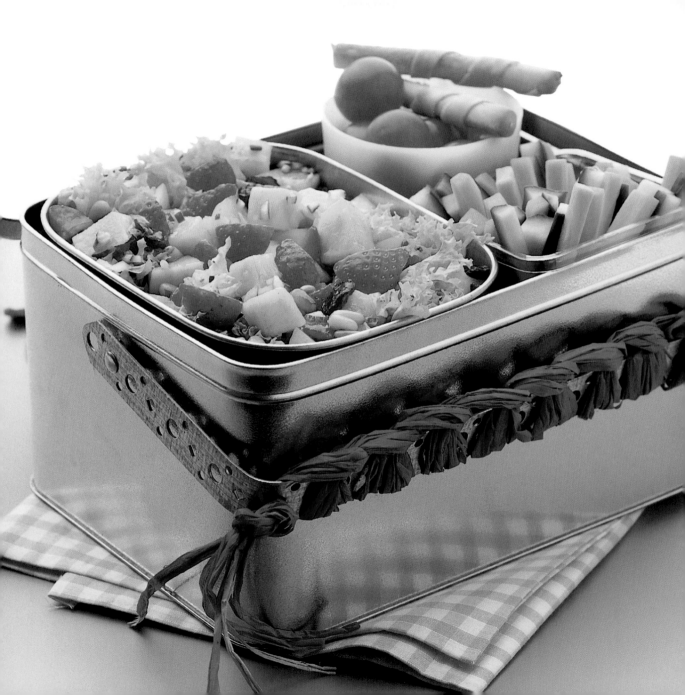

# orzo salad

Orzo pasta is shaped like rice. If you can't find it, try mini pasta shells.

⌣ **Makes 1 portion**
*¼ cup orzo*
*2 tablespoons cooked frozen peas*
*¼ cup canned corn*
*½ cup diced cooked chicken*

**Dressing**
*1 tablespoon mayonnaise*
*1 tablespoon sour cream or Greek-style yogurt*
*1 teaspoon water*
*½ teaspoon white wine vinegar*
*1½ teaspoons snipped fresh chives*

Cook the orzo according to the package directions. Drain and mix with the peas, corn, and chicken.

Whisk together all the dressing ingredients and toss with the salad.

# chinese noodle salad

⌣ **Makes 1 to 2 portions**
*2 ounces chow mein noodles*
*½ cup shredded cooked chicken*
*1 small carrot, peeled and cut into very thin strips*
*1 small red bell pepper, cut into very thin strips*

**Soy dressing**
*1 tablespoon sunflower or canola oil*
*1½ teaspoons soy sauce*
*1 teaspoon honey*
*2 teaspoons rice wine vinegar*

*1 scallion, thinly sliced*
*a little fresh coriander, chopped (optional)*

Cook the noodles according to the package directions, then rinse in a sieve. Mix together with the chicken, carrot, and bell pepper.

Whisk together the dressing ingredients and toss with the noodles. Garnish with the scallion and some coriander (if using).

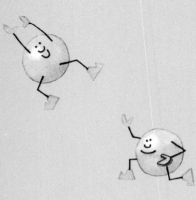

# cheat's chicken and potato salad

You could use ham, turkey, or sausage instead of chicken.

🥣 **Makes 2 portions**
*1 cup store-bought potato salad*
*½ cup halved cherry tomatoes*
*¾ cup diced cooked chicken*
*1 large scallion, sliced*
*snipped fresh chives, to serve (optional)*

Simply mix together all the ingredients. If your potato salad already includes onion, leave out the scallion.

---

**LUNCH BOX LOWDOWN**

It is likely that your child will only accept food that he feels comfortable eating in the school dining room. Most children are greatly influenced by peer pressure, and just because your child will eat raw cauliflower with a dip at home, it doesn't mean he will be comfortable eating it at school. The trick is to find foods that suit your nutritional standards and are also acceptable among your child's social set.

---

# chicken superfood salad

Toast the sunflower seeds in a dry frying pan, stirring occasionally, until golden.

🥣 **Makes 2 portions**
*1 cup fusilli pasta*
*¾ cup small broccoli florets*
*½ cup shredded cooked chicken*
*3 tablespoons sunflower seeds, toasted*
*1 tomato, seeded and cut into strips*

**Dressing (or use pesto dressing on page 74)**
*2 tablespoons olive oil*
*2 teaspoons balsamic vinegar*
*½ teaspoon honey*

*salt and freshly ground black pepper*

Cook the pasta according to the package directions, adding the broccoli for the last 3 minutes of the cooking time. Drain and rinse under cold water and drain thoroughly. Transfer to a large bowl and add the chicken, sunflower seeds, and tomato.

To make the dressing, either whisk the ingredients together or put them in a jam jar, seal, and shake well to mix. Pour over the salad and season to taste.

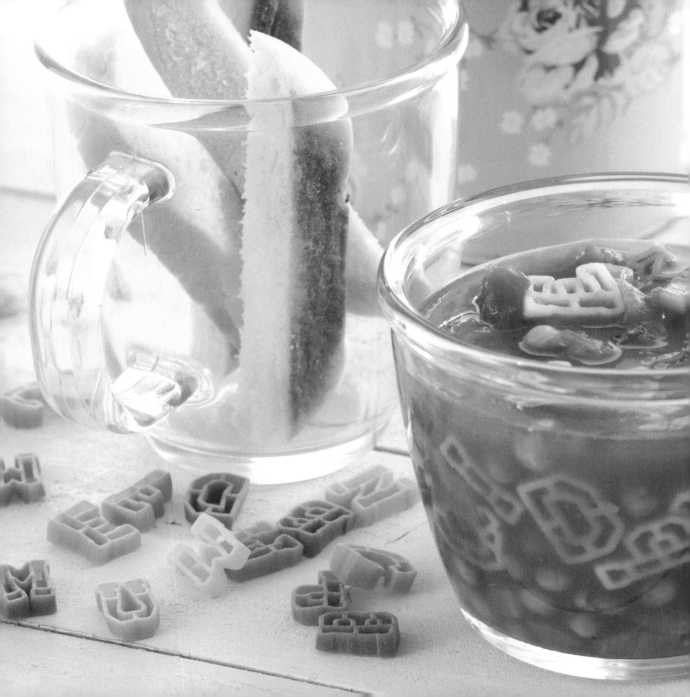

# super soups

When the weather gets cold, your child may welcome something hot for lunch. Fill a small thermos with one of these tasty soups.

*alphabet minestrone (see page 92)*

# cauliflower cheese soup

⌒ **Makes 6 portions**
❊ **Suitable for freezing**
*1 tablespoon butter*
*1 large onion, finely chopped*
*1 large cauliflower, leaves removed, cut into florets*
*1 large potato, peeled and cut into chunks*
*3 cups vegetable broth*
*1¾ cups milk*
*salt and freshly ground black pepper*
*½ cup grated sharp Cheddar cheese*

Melt the butter in a large saucepan. Sauté the onion for about 5 minutes, until softened but not colored. Add the cauliflower, potato, broth, milk, and seasonings. Bring to a boil, then reduce the heat and leave to simmer uncovered for about 30 minutes until the vegetables are soft.

Remove from the heat and stir in the cheese until melted. Whiz in a food processor to make a thick, creamy soup.

> ### LUNCH BOX LOWDOWN
> Any of the soups in this chapter can be frozen in individual containers. Thaw a portion overnight, then heat it up in the morning and pour it into a thermos to keep it hot until lunchtime.

# homemade tomato soup

Homemade tomato soup is a favorite with everyone and this one is particularly delicious.

⌒ **Makes 5 portions**
❊ **Suitable for freezing**
*1½ tablespoons olive oil*
*1 onion, chopped*
*2 carrots, peeled and chopped*
*one 14.5-ounce can diced tomatoes*
*1 tablespoon tomato paste*
*2 teaspoons garlic puree,*
*    or 1 large clove garlic, crushed*
*½ teaspoon superfine sugar*
*1½ cups vegetable or chicken broth*
*1 bay leaf*
*salt and freshly ground black pepper*
*3 tablespoons heavy cream (optional)*
*2 tablespoons torn fresh basil leaves (optional)*

Warm the olive oil in a saucepan over low heat, add the onion and carrots, and sauté for 5 minutes. Add the tomatoes, tomato paste, garlic puree, sugar, broth, bay leaf, and seasonings and bring to a boil. Reduce the heat, cover, and simmer for 20 minutes. Remove the bay leaf.

Transfer to a blender and blend until smooth. Return the soup to the pan, add the cream and basil (if using), and reheat.

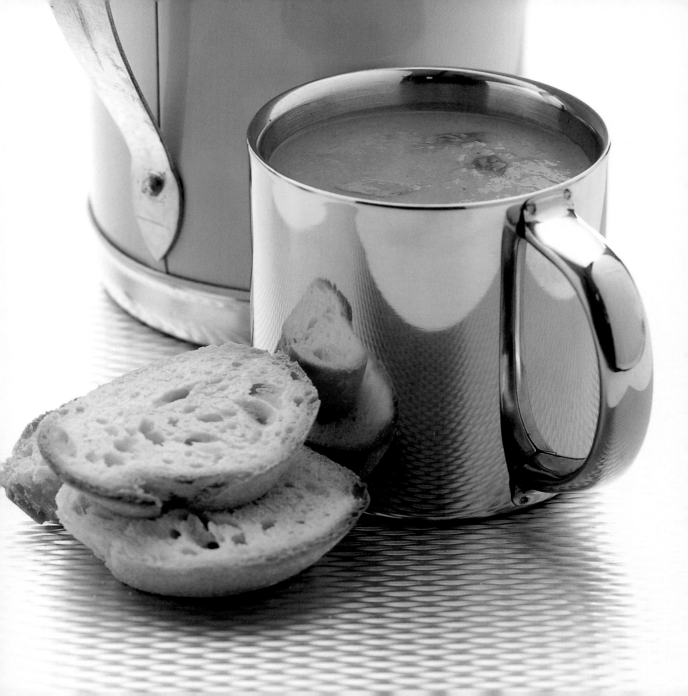

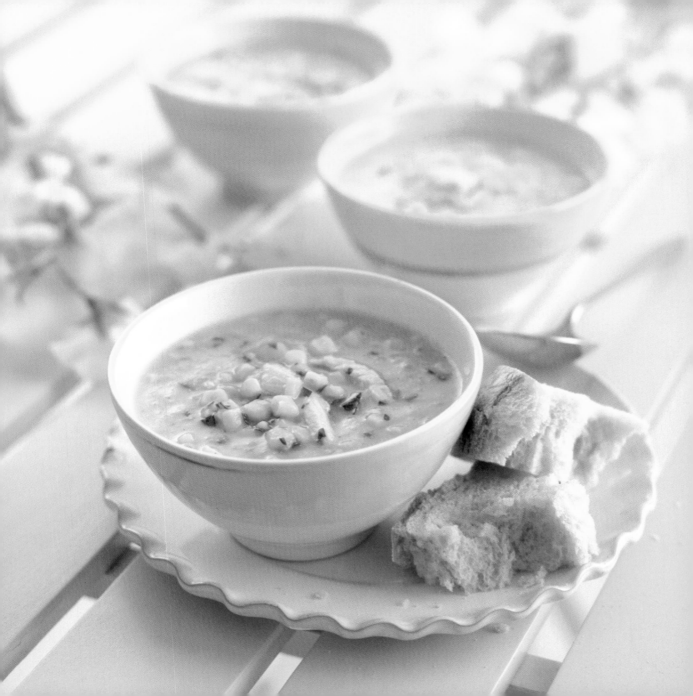

# chicken and corn chowder

My three children love this soup, and it's very quick and easy to prepare and a complete meal in a bowl. Include this in a thermos in your child's lunch box when the weather gets cold. For a vegetarian version, leave out the shredded chicken and use vegetable broth. As well as being rich in antioxidants and minerals, corn is packed with fiber to help keep your child regular.

▽ **Makes 4 portions**
❋ **Suitable for freezing**
*1 tablespoon butter*
*1 large shallot, finely chopped*
*1 medium potato, peeled and cut into ¹/₂-inch dice*
*one 14-ounce can corn, drained*
*2³/₄ cups good-quality chicken broth*
*6 tablespoons heavy cream*
*salt and freshly ground black pepper*
*¹/₂ cup shredded cooked chicken*
*1 tablespoon chopped parsley (optional)*

Melt the butter in a large saucepan over low heat and sauté the shallot for 5 minutes or until soft. Add the potato, corn, and broth, then bring to a simmer and cook until the potato is soft. Blend half of the mixture until smooth, then return to the pan and stir in the cream. Season to taste. Stir in the shredded chicken. If you wish, serve sprinkled with a little chopped parsley.

# chicken soup with rice

This is the most delicious soup and really good to make when you have leftover roast chicken.

▽ **Makes 4 portions**
❋ **Suitable for freezing**
*¹/₃ cup rice*
*¹/₂ medium onion, chopped*
*1 tablespoon olive oil*
*1 medium carrot, peeled and diced*
*2 cups good-quality chicken broth*
*¹/₂ teaspoon fresh thyme leaves*
*¹/₃ cup frozen peas*
*¹/₃ cup canned corn*
*1 cup shredded cooked chicken*
*salt and freshly ground black pepper*

Cook the rice according to the package directions. Gently sauté the onion in the oil for about 5 minutes. Add the carrot, broth, and thyme and simmer for 4 to 5 minutes until the carrot is soft. Add the peas and corn and simmer for 3 minutes more. Add the chicken to the soup, together with the rice, and simmer for 2 minutes to reheat. Season with a little salt and pepper.

**LUNCH BOX LOWDOWN**
To improve heat retention, rinse the thermos with hot water before pouring in hot soup.

# alphabet minestrone

◯ Makes 3 to 4 portions
❄ Suitable for freezing

2 tablespoons olive oil
1 onion, diced
1 clove garlic, crushed
1 small carrot, peeled and diced
½ small celery stalk, diced
half a 14.5-ounce can plum tomatoes, drained and chopped
1 tablespoon tomato paste
4 cups chicken or vegetable broth
¾ cup alphabet pasta
1 bay leaf
sprig of fresh thyme or pinch of dried thyme
1 cup frozen peas
salt and freshly ground black pepper
freshly grated Parmesan cheese (optional)

**This minestrone soup is easy to prepare and takes less than 20 minutes.**

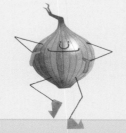

Heat the olive oil in a large saucepan and gently sauté the onion and garlic for 5 minutes. Add the carrot and celery and cook for a further 5 minutes. Add the tomatoes, tomato paste, broth, pasta, bay leaf, and thyme. Bring to a boil, reduce the heat, and simmer for 6 minutes.

Add the peas and bring back to a boil. Reduce the heat and simmer for a further 3 minutes. Remove the bay leaf. Season to taste and sprinkle some freshly grated Parmesan on top (if using).

(see photograph on pages 86–87)

**LUNCH BOX LOWDOWN**
Soups are great for warming you up on a cold day, but there are plenty of other meals that you can put into a wide-mouthed thermos. Why not try pasta shapes with Bolognese sauce, or chicken and vegetable stir-fries?

# minestrone soup with beans

⌒ **Makes 8 to 10 portions**
❋ **Suitable for freezing**
*2 tablespoons olive oil*
*1 carrot, peeled and finely diced*
*1 celery stalk, finely diced*
*1 red onion, finely diced*
*1 clove garlic, crushed*
*5 ripe plum tomatoes, peeled, seeded, and roughly chopped*
   *(or one 14.5-ounce can diced tomatoes)*
*1 tablespoon tomato paste*
*8 cups chicken broth*
*1 small head cabbage, finely sliced*
*8 basil leaves, torn*
*⅔ cup small pasta shapes or broken spaghetti*
*one 15-ounce can Great Northern or cannellini beans or baked beans*
*salt and freshly ground black pepper*
*freshly grated Parmesan cheese, to serve*

Heat the olive oil in a large saucepan. Add the carrot, celery, onion, and garlic and sauté for 10 minutes, stirring occasionally. Add the tomatoes, tomato paste, and broth. Bring to a boil, reduce the heat, and simmer for 15 minutes.

Stir in the cabbage, basil, pasta, and beans and simmer for 15 to 18 minutes until the pasta is tender. Season to taste.

Pack some grated Parmesan in a separate container for your child to add at lunchtime.

**All beans are rich in protein, vitamins, and minerals.**

## TOP SNACKING TIP
Make sure your children eat their after-school snack as far in advance as possible of their main meal so they don't spoil their appetites.

# chicken noodle soup

○ **Makes 4 to 6 portions**
❊ **Suitable for freezing**
*1 tablespoon olive oil*
*1 small onion, chopped*
*1 medium carrot, peeled and diced*
*¼ red bell pepper, diced*
*6 cups chicken broth*
*⅔ cup mini pasta shells*
*1 tablespoon tomato paste*
*1 teaspoon fresh thyme leaves*
*½ cup shredded cooked chicken*
*½ cup canned corn*
*⅔ cup frozen peas*

Heat the oil in a large saucepan and sauté the onion for 10 minutes or until soft. Add the carrot and bell pepper and cook for 5 minutes. Add the chicken broth and bring to a boil, then stir in the pasta, tomato paste, and thyme. Bring back to a boil, reduce the heat, and simmer for 10 minutes. Add the chicken, corn, and peas and cook for another 2 minutes.

> **LUNCH BOX LOWDOWN**
> Children tend to arrive home from school famished. Try to set aside a few minutes to prepare some healthy snacks, rather than letting them have cookies and a package of potato chips.

# thai-style chicken soup

This easy-to-prepare soup is ready in about 10 minutes and is almost a meal in itself.

○ **Makes 4 portions**
❊ **Suitable for freezing**
*1 tablespoon olive oil*
*½ cup chopped onion*
*1 clove garlic, crushed*
*½ red chile, finely chopped*
*1 small skinless, boneless chicken breast,*
*    cut into thin strips*
*1 cup broccoli florets*
*3 cups chicken broth*
*1¼ cups coconut milk*
*salt and freshly ground black pepper*
*¼ cup rice, cooked according to package directions,*
*    or 1⅓ cups cooked rice*

Heat the oil in a saucepan and sauté the onion, garlic, and chile for 2 minutes. Add the strips of chicken and sauté for 2 minutes more. Add the broccoli and chicken broth and bring to a boil. Reduce the heat and simmer for 4 minutes. Stir in the coconut milk and simmer for 2 minutes. Season to taste and stir in the cooked rice.

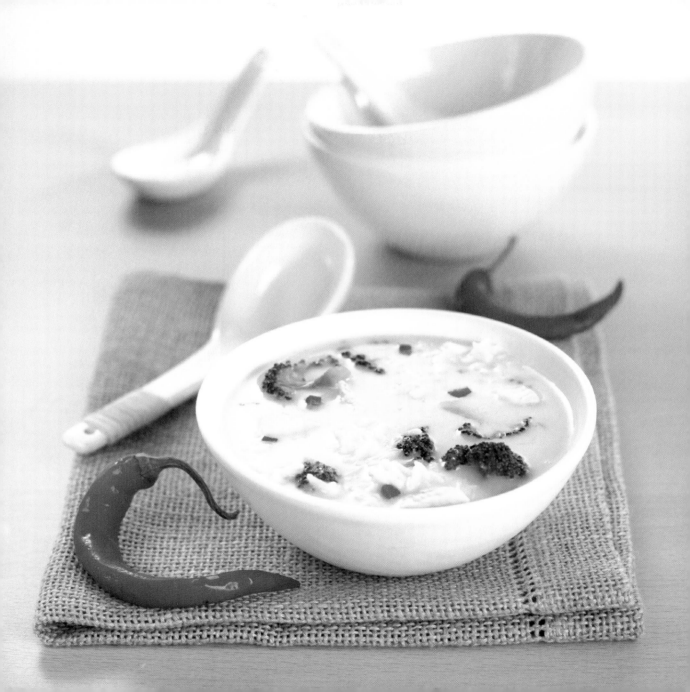

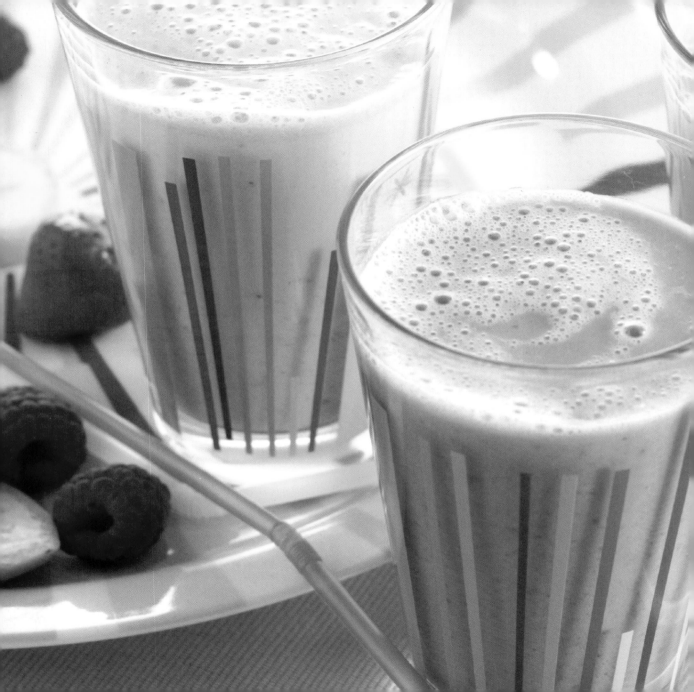

# sweet
# sensations

Nothing beats the taste of home-baked cookies and muffins, and here
you'll find quick and easy recipes for children to try themselves.
To keep those lunch boxes looking healthy, you will also find
many tempting recipes and ideas for fresh fruit.

*fruit smoothies (see page 122)*

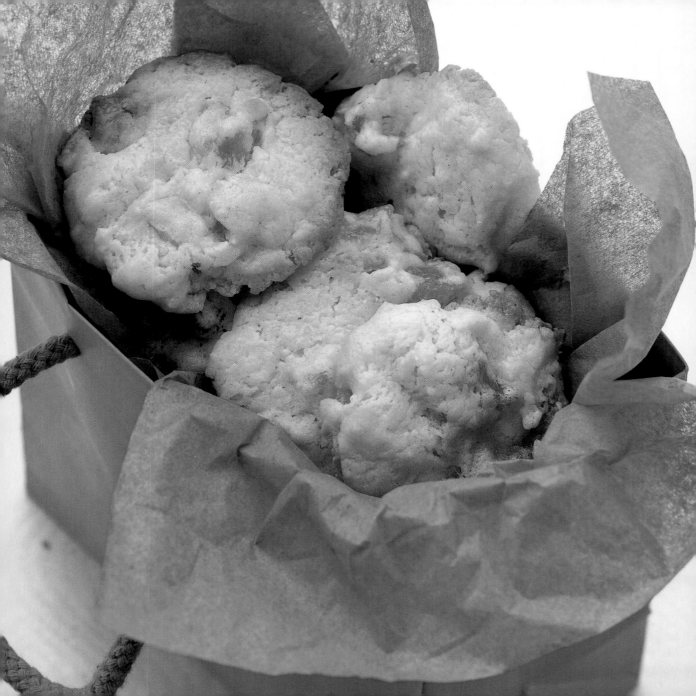

# annabel's apricot cookies

These are my son Nicholas's favorite cookies. They are a rather unusual but totally irresistible combination of dried apricots, cream cheese, and white chocolate.

◯ **Makes about 18 cookies**
❄ **Suitable for freezing**
*8 tablespoons (1 stick) unsalted butter*
*4 ounces cream cheese*
*1/2 cup superfine sugar*
*1/2 cup all-purpose flour*
*1/4 cup chopped dried apricots*
*1/2 cup white chocolate chips or*
*    chopped white chocolate*

Preheat the oven to 350°F. Line some baking sheets with parchment or other baking paper (unless using nonstick).

In a large mixing bowl, cream together the butter and cream cheese. Add the sugar and beat until fluffy. Gradually add the flour, then fold in the apricots and chocolate. The dough will be quite soft—don't worry!

Drop heaping teaspoons of the mixture onto the baking sheets and bake for about 15 minutes until lightly golden. Allow the cookies to cool and harden for a few minutes, then transfer to a wire rack.

# my favorite chocolate chip cookies

◯ **Makes about 36 cookies**
❄ **Suitable for freezing**
*1 cup packed light brown sugar*
*1/2 cup granulated sugar*
*8 tablespoons (1 stick) unsalted butter*
*1/2 cup vegetable shortening*
*1 1/2 teaspoons vanilla extract*
*1 egg*
*1 3/4 cups all-purpose flour*
*1 teaspoon baking soda*
*1/2 teaspoon salt*
*6 ounces white or semisweet chocolate,*
*    broken into pieces*
*1/3 cup sunflower seeds or chopped pecans*
*    (optional)*

Preheat the oven to 375°F. Line some baking sheets with parchment or other baking paper (unless using nonstick).

In an electric mixer, cream together the sugars, butter, and shortening and beat until light and fluffy. Add the vanilla and egg and blend well. Then mix in the flour, baking soda, and salt, followed by the chocolate and sunflower seeds (if using). Using floured hands, form the mixture into walnut-size balls and place them about 2 inches apart on the baking sheets.

Bake for 8 to 10 minutes until lightly golden. Leave to cool for a few minutes, then transfer to a wire rack.

# energy bars

◯ **Makes 8 bars**

6 tablespoons (¾ stick) unsalted butter

½ cup packed light brown sugar

¼ cup light corn syrup or golden syrup, such as
    Lyle's

½ teaspoon salt

1½ cups quick-cooking oats

1 cup cornflakes

2 tablespoons sunflower seeds

⅓ cup raisins

Preheat the oven to 350°F. Line an 8-inch square baking pan with parchment or other baking paper.

In a saucepan, melt together the butter, sugar, syrup, and salt. In a bowl, combine all the dry ingredients, then stir in the butter and syrup mixture until well coated.

Spoon the mixture into the pan and press down with a potato masher. Bake for 18 to 20 minutes. When cool, store in the fridge. Cut into bars before serving.

> ### TOP SNACKING TIP
> Why not take your children shopping to choose their own snacks? For every four healthy snacks they select, allow them to choose a less healthy treat.

# oat, raisin, and sunflower seed cookies

This is one of my favorite cookie recipes. These cookies make a tasty and nutritious snack at any time of the day. As they are egg free, they are ideal for anyone who is allergic to eggs.

◯ **Makes about 14 cookies**

❄ **Suitable for freezing**

6 tablespoons (¾ stick) unsalted butter

½ cup packed light brown sugar

1 teaspoon vanilla extract

½ cup raisins

¼ cup sunflower seeds

½ cup all-purpose flour

1 cup quick-cooking oats

¼ teaspoon baking soda

½ teaspoon salt

Preheat the oven to 350°F.

Cream together the butter and sugar until light and fluffy. Add the remaining ingredients and stir until completely combined. Shape into walnut-size balls and flatten them onto a nonstick baking tray with your hand. Bake for about 15 minutes until golden. The cookies will be soft but will harden a little when cooled.

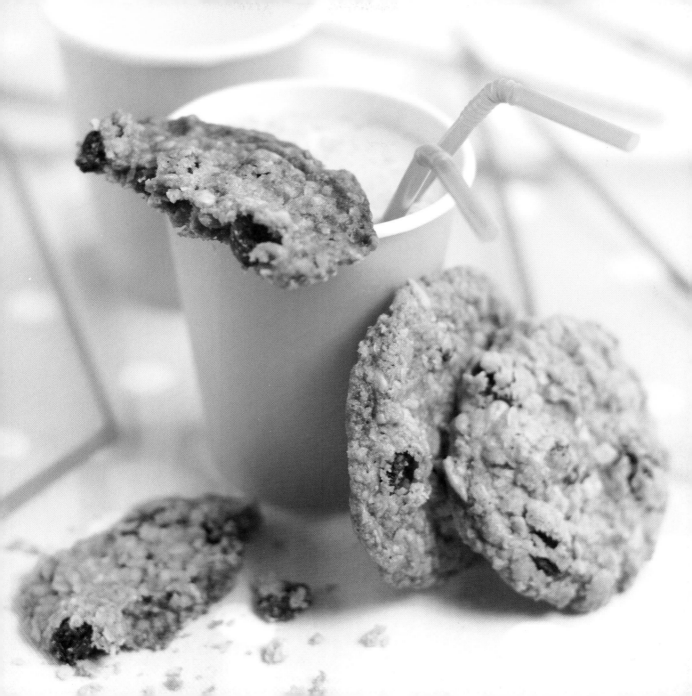

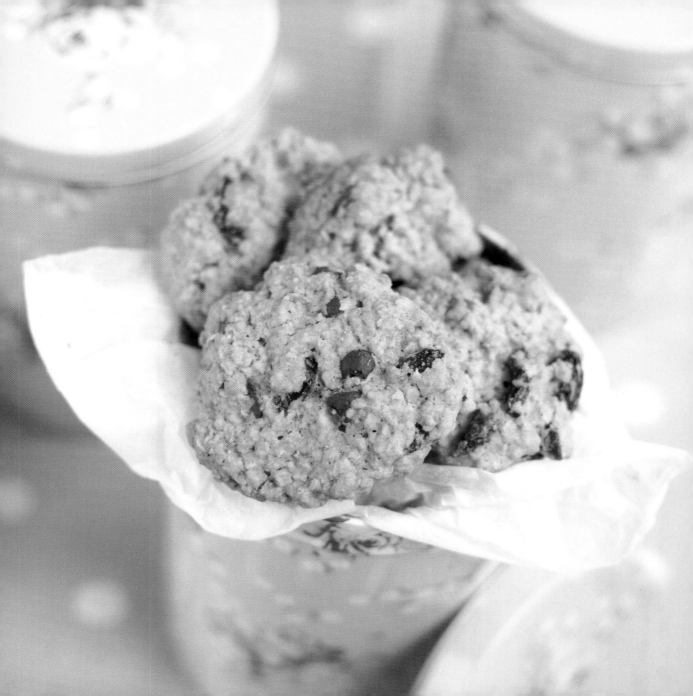

# loaded oatmeal cookies

I tend to make these without pecans when preparing them for children. If you don't have chocolate chips, use chopped chocolate.

� **Makes about 24 cookies**
*4 tablespoons (¹/₂ stick) unsalted butter, softened*
*¹/₄ cup vegetable shortening, softened*
*³/₄ cup packed light brown sugar*
*1 egg*
*1 teaspoon vanilla extract*
*²/₃ cup all-purpose flour*
*1 teaspoon baking powder*
*¹/₂ teaspoon salt*
*1¹/₂ cups quick-cooking oats*
*¹/₃ cup chocolate chips*
*¹/₂ cup raisins*
*¹/₂ cup chopped pecans (optional)*

Preheat the oven to 350°F. Grease two large baking sheets.

Cream the butter, shortening, and sugar until pale and fluffy. Beat in the egg, then the vanilla. In a large bowl, sift together the flour, baking powder, salt, and oats. Fold into the butter mixture. Stir in the chocolate chips, raisins, and pecans (if using).

Drop heaping tablespoons of the mixture onto the baking sheets, spaced about 2 inches apart. Bake for 12 to 15 minutes until lightly browned around the edges. Leave for 5 minutes, then transfer to a wire rack using a spatula. Allow to cool completely.

# chewy oatmeal raisin cookies

These cookies are so easy to make and they are hard to resist and good for you, too—oats and raisins are a great source of energy.

⌣ **Makes about 24 cookies**
❄ **Suitable for freezing**
*9 tablespoons (1 stick plus 1 tablespoon) unsalted butter*
*¹/₂ cup superfine sugar*
*¹/₂ cup packed light brown sugar*
*1 egg*
*1 teaspoon vanilla extract*
*1 cup all-purpose flour*
*1 teaspoon baking powder*
*¹/₂ teaspoon pumpkin pie spice*
*¹/₂ teaspoon salt*
*1 cup quick-cooking oats*
*³/₄ cup raisins*

Preheat the oven to 350°F. Grease or line two large baking sheets with parchment or other baking paper.

Put the butter and sugars in a bowl and beat until light and fluffy. Beat in the egg and vanilla. In a separate bowl, mix together the flour, baking powder, spice, salt, and oats, then stir into the butter mixture. Finally, stir in the raisins.

Shape the mixture into walnut-size balls and place on the baking sheets, spacing them out well. Flatten with your fingers, then bake for about 15 minutes until the edges are lightly golden. Leave to cool for a few minutes, then transfer to a wire rack. Store in a sealed container.

# power-packed oat bars with cranberries, apricots, and pumpkin seeds

These delicious energy bars are packed full of nutritious ingredients.

◯ **Makes 8 bars**
7 tablespoons unsalted butter
½ cup packed light brown sugar
5 tablespoons light corn syrup or golden syrup, such as Lyle's
½ teaspoon salt
1½ cups quick-cooking oats
¼ cup chopped dried apple
¼ cup chopped dried apricots
¼ cup dried cranberries
¼ cup pumpkin seeds
2 tablespoons sunflower seeds
¼ cup dried coconut

Preheat the oven to 350°F. Line and grease an 8-inch square baking pan. In a saucepan, melt together the butter, sugar, syrup, and salt. In a bowl, combine the oats, dried apple, apricots, and cranberries, pumpkin and sunflower seeds, and coconut. Stir in the butter mixture. Spoon the mixture into the pan and press down with a potato masher to compress and level the surface. Bake for 18 to 20 minutes. Allow to cool for 15 minutes; cut into bars with a sharp knife. Allow to cool completely before lifting from the pan. Store in the fridge.

# maple pecan bars

These bars are delicious. They are quite crumbly; if made with maple syrup rather than corn or golden syrup, they're not as sticky as other bar cookies.

◯ **Makes 8 bars**
1 tablespoon unsalted butter
½ cup packed light brown sugar
¼ cup maple syrup or light corn syrup or golden syrup, such as Lyle's
1½ cups quick-cooking oats
½ teaspoon salt
¼ cup raisins
¼ cup chopped dried apple
⅓ cup dried cranberries
½ cup chopped pecans
1 large egg, lightly beaten

Preheat the oven to 350°F. Line an 8-inch square pan with baking paper such as parchment.

Put the butter, sugar, and syrup in a saucepan and melt together over low heat. Put the oats, salt, raisins, dried apple and cranberries, and pecans in a large bowl. Pour in the butter mixture, stir in the egg, and mix thoroughly.

Transfer to the pan and bake for 25 to 30 minutes until firm in the center.

Leave in the pan for 10 minutes. Using a sharp knife, mark into eight bars, then allow to cool completely before lifting from the pan. Store in the fridge.

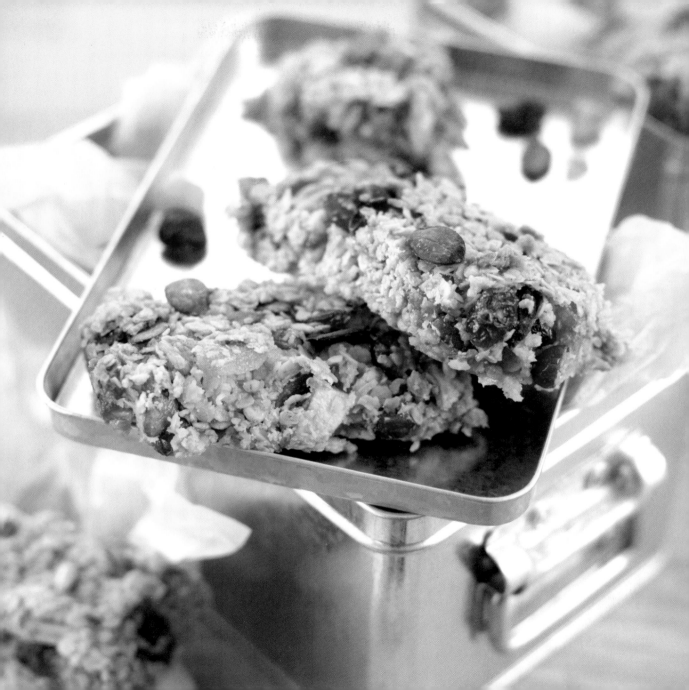

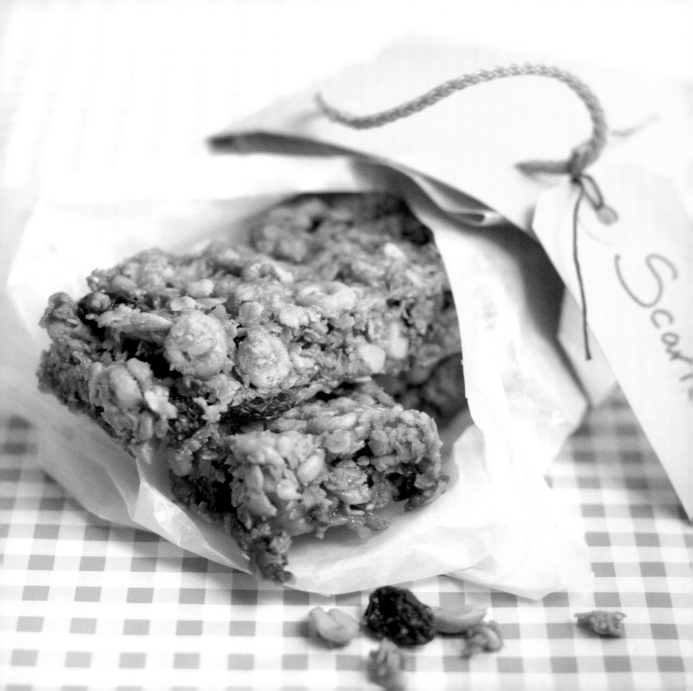

Trail mix is a snack food commonly used in activities like hiking, backpacking, and mountaineering. It usually consists of a mixture of nuts, seeds, and dried fruits such as raisins and cranberries. It is energy rich and has a high content of vitamins and minerals. Try pumpkin seeds instead of nuts, or dried cranberries rather than chocolate chips.

## LUNCH BOX LOWDOWN

With some schools banning chocolate from packed lunches, cereal bars are the obvious substitute. However, do check the label before you buy; some cereal bars are more than 40 percent sugar and more than 30 percent fat. Also, while sugar eaten in a bowl of cereal tends to get washed away by the milk, in sticky cereal bars sugar sticks to the teeth, causing maximum damage.

# trail mix bars

◯ **Makes 8 bars**

4 tablespoons (½ stick) unsalted butter
3 tablespoons honey
1⅓ cups quick-cooking oats
½ cup packed light brown sugar
¾ cup Cheerios
¼ cup raisins
¼ cup salted peanuts or pumpkin seeds
¼ cup milk chocolate chips
¼ cup sunflower seeds
¼ teaspoon salt

Preheat the oven to 325°F. Line an 8-inch square pan with parchment or other baking paper and lightly grease.

Put the butter and honey in a small saucepan and heat gently until the butter has melted. Set aside to cool.

Put the remaining ingredients in a large bowl and stir to combine. Add the cooled butter mixture and mix well. Transfer to the prepared pan and press down firmly with a potato masher. Bake for 30 minutes or until the center is just firm to the touch.

Allow to cool for 15 minutes, then mark into eight bars, using a sharp knife. Allow to cool completely before lifting from the pan. Store in an airtight container.

# flourless peanut butter cookies

▽ **Makes 18 to 20 cookies**
❋ **Suitable for freezing**
*1 cup smooth peanut butter (room temperature)*
*³⁄₄ cup superfine sugar*
*1 large egg*
*¹⁄₄ teaspoon baking soda*
*large pinch of salt*
*1 cup milk chocolate chips or chopped milk chocolate*

Preheat the oven to 350°F.

Put the peanut butter, sugar, egg, baking soda, and salt in a large bowl and mix with a wooden spoon until thoroughly combined. Mix in the chocolate chips.

Take rounded tablespoons of the mixture and roll into balls. It helps to dip the spoon in water after every couple of cookies. Place the balls on baking sheets, spacing them 2 inches apart. Flatten the balls slightly with your fingers and bake for 12 to 15 minutes. The cookies should spread out during cooking and have a final thickness of around ¹⁄₄ inch. They will have a slightly cracked surface.

Leave the cookies on the baking sheets for 10 minutes to cool, then carefully transfer to a wire rack using a spatula. Allow to cool completely, then store in an airtight container for up to three days. If frozen, thaw the cookies by spreading them out on a baking sheet or plate at room temperature for 30 minutes.

**These cookies taste so good, you would never know that they're made without flour.**

### LUNCH BOX LOWDOWN
You don't always have to give your child fruit juice in his lunch box. A bottle of water is just as good— it's the most thirst-quenching drink and it won't spoil his appetite.

# apple and carrot muffins with maple syrup

○ **Makes 12 muffins**
❄ **Suitable for freezing**
*1 cup whole wheat flour*
*¼ cup sugar*
*¼ cup nonfat dry milk*
*1½ teaspoons baking powder*
*½ teaspoon ground cinnamon*
*½ teaspoon ground ginger*
*½ teaspoon salt*
*½ cup vegetable oil*
*3 tablespoons maple syrup*
*1 tablespoon honey*
*2 eggs, lightly beaten*
*½ teaspoon vanilla extract*
*1 large apple, peeled and grated*
*1 medium carrot, peeled and grated*
*½ cup raisins*

Preheat the oven to 350°F. Line a muffin pan with paper cups.

Combine the seven dry ingredients in a mixing bowl. In a separate bowl, mix the oil, maple syrup, honey, eggs, and vanilla. Beat lightly with a wire whisk until blended. Add the apple, carrot, and raisins and stir well. Fold in the dry ingredients until just combined, but don't overmix.

Spoon the mixture into the paper cups until two-thirds full. Bake for 20 to 25 minutes. Allow to cool for a few minutes, then remove from the pan and cool on a wire rack.

# mini chocolate chip muffins

Mini muffins are just the right size for small children and these are delicious. They are easy to make and older children will have fun making them themselves.

○ **Makes 32 mini muffins**
❄ **Suitable for freezing**
*1 cup self-rising flour*
*2 tablespoons cocoa powder*
*half an 8-ounce tub soft margarine, or*
  *1 stick unsalted butter*
*½ cup superfine sugar*
*2 eggs, lightly beaten*
*½ teaspoon grated orange zest*
*⅓ cup dark chocolate chips*

Preheat the oven to 350°F. Line three mini muffin pans with paper cups.

Sift together the flour and cocoa and, in a separate bowl, cream together the margarine and sugar. Add the eggs to the creamed mixture a little at a time, adding a tablespoon of the flour mixture with the second egg. Mix in the remaining flour and cocoa until just blended. Stir in the orange zest and chocolate chips. Don't overmix. Spoon the mixture into the paper cups until two-thirds full.

Bake the muffins for 12 to 15 minutes until a toothpick comes out clean. Allow to cool for a few minutes, then remove from the pan and cool on a wire rack.

# apple and raisin bran muffins

Complex carbohydrates satisfy the appetite longer than refined carbohydrates do and provide sustained energy. These delicious muffins will give your child a real energy boost at any time.

## ▽ Makes 10 muffins

1/2 cup whole wheat flour
1 1/2 teaspoons baking powder
1 teaspoon ground ginger
1 teaspoon pumpkin pie spice
3/4 cup wheat bran
3/4 cup packed light brown sugar *(1/4 c !)*
1 large apple, peeled and grated
3/4 cup raisins
1/2 cup vegetable oil
2 eggs, beaten          *1 tsp vanilla*
2 tablespoons honey
1 tablespoon maple syrup
2 tablespoons milk

Preheat the oven to 350°F. Line a muffin pan with paper cups.

Mix together the flour, baking powder, ginger, spice, wheat bran, and sugar. Add the apple and raisins. In a separate bowl, mix the vegetable oil, eggs, honey, maple syrup, and milk. Pour into the flour mixture and stir until just combined.

Spoon the mixture into the paper cups and bake for about 25 minutes until golden.

# date and raisin muffins

## ▽ Makes 8 muffins

1 cup dates, pitted and chopped
4 tablespoons (1/2 stick) unsalted butter
1/3 cup packed dark brown sugar
1/3 cup milk
1 egg, beaten
1/2 teaspoon vanilla extract
3/4 cup all-purpose flour
1/2 teaspoon baking soda
1/2 teaspoon baking powder
1/4 teaspoon salt
1/4 cup raisins

Bring 1/2 cup water to a boil in a saucepan. Add the dates and simmer for 10 to 15 minutes until the dates are very soft and all the water has been absorbed. Set aside to cool for 10 minutes.

Preheat the oven to 350°F. Line a muffin pan with paper cups.

Melt the butter in a saucepan and stir in the sugar. Allow to cool slightly, then mix in the dates, milk, egg, and vanilla. Sift together the flour, baking soda, baking powder, and salt, then stir in the raisins. Add the date mixture to the dry ingredients and stir until just combined.

Spoon in enough muffin batter to half fill each paper cup. Bake for 18 to 20 minutes until risen and slightly firm to the touch. Leave to cool on a wire rack.

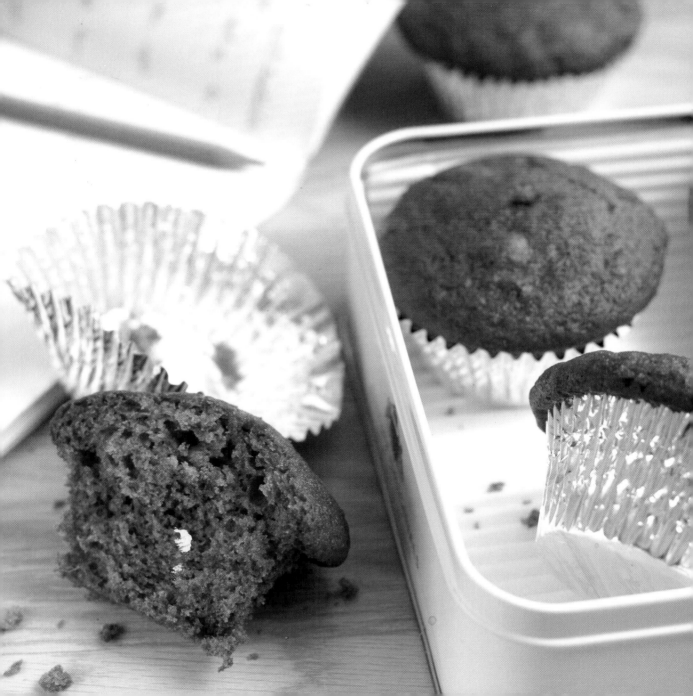

# carrot and pineapple muffins

These are probably my favorite muffins. They are like miniature carrot cakes and are lovely and moist. You can make them with or without the icing.

⬭ **Makes 12 muffins**
3/4 cup all-purpose flour
3/4 cup whole wheat flour
1 teaspoon baking powder
1/2 teaspoon baking soda
1 1/2 teaspoons ground cinnamon
1/2 teaspoon salt
1 cup vegetable oil
1/2 cup superfine sugar
2 eggs
1 large carrot, peeled and finely grated
one 8-ounce can crushed pineapple, semi-drained
3/4 cup raisins
1/3 cup chopped pecans (optional)

***Cream cheese icing***
6 ounces cream cheese
1/2 cup confectioners' sugar, sifted
1/2 vanilla bean

Preheat the oven to 350°F. Line a muffin pan with paper cups.

Sift together the flours, baking powder, baking soda, cinnamon, and salt and mix well. In a separate bowl, beat together the oil, sugar, and eggs. Add the carrot, pineapple, raisins, and pecans (if using). Gradually add the flour mixture, beating until the ingredients are just combined.

Pour the mixture into the paper cups and bake for 25 minutes. Allow the muffins to cool for a few minutes, then transfer to a wire rack.

To make the icing, beat the cream cheese together with the sugar. Split the vanilla bean and scrape out the tiny black seeds. Stir these into the icing and spread over the tops of the muffins.

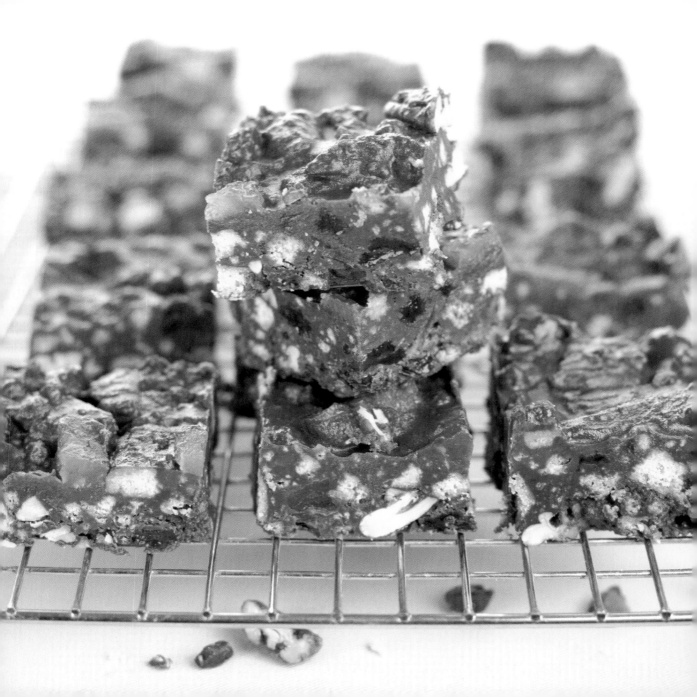

# no-cook chocolate cookie squares

**This is a slight variation on the classic chocolate cookie squares—I use ginger snaps and Rice Krispies as well as graham crackers.**

◯ **Makes 12 squares**

*1 cup ginger snaps*

*5 sheets graham crackers*

*4 ounces milk chocolate*

*4 ounces dark chocolate*

*5 tablespoons light corn syrup or golden syrup, such as Lyle's*

*6 tablespoons (¾ stick) unsalted butter*

*8 dried apricots, finely chopped*

*¼ cup halved raisins*

*1 cup Rice Krispies*

Lightly grease and line a shallow 8-inch square pan.

Break the ginger snaps and graham crackers into pieces, place in a plastic bag, and crush with a rolling pin to form coarse crumbs.

Melt the chocolates, syrup, and butter in a heatproof bowl over a pan of simmering water. Stir in the crumbs until well coated. Add the apricots and raisins and mix, and finally stir in the Rice Krispies.

Spoon the mixture into the prepared pan, and level the surface by pressing down with a potato masher. Allow to cool, chill in the fridge for 1 hour, and cut into squares. Store in the fridge.

> **LUNCH BOX LOWDOWN**
> Communicate with your child; ask him what he enjoyed in his lunch box today. Look at what comes back untouched and ask, without being defensive, why it wasn't eaten and if there are any foods that other children bring to school that he would like to try.

## chocolate and apricot Rice Krispies squares

These are always popular, and older children love to make them. They can also be made with white chocolate and you could add some chopped pecans.

◯ **Makes 12 squares**
*6 tablespoons (¾ stick) unsalted butter*
*¼ cup light corn syrup or golden syrup, such as Lyle's*
*2½ ounces bittersweet chocolate, broken into pieces*
*1 cup Rice Krispies*
*1 cup quick-cooking oats*
*8 dried apricots, finely chopped (and/or mango)*

Lightly grease and line a shallow 8-inch square pan.

Put the butter, syrup, and chocolate into a small saucepan and melt over low heat. Mix together the Rice Krispies, oats, and chopped apricots and stir into the syrup mixture.

Spoon the mixture into the prepared pan, and level the surface by pressing down with a potato masher. Allow to cool, chill in the fridge for 1 hour, and cut into squares.

## exotic fruit, white chocolate, and cereal cupcakes

These are quick and easy for children to make themselves and are a lovely lunch box treat. Oats and dried fruits provide a good source of energy to keep your child going through the afternoon.

◯ **Makes 12 cupcakes**
*1½ cups quick-cooking oats*
*2 cups Rice Krispies*
*⅔ cup chopped mixed exotic dried fruits (such as papaya, mango, and pineapple)*
*½ cup chopped pecans*
*8 tablespoons (1 stick) unsalted butter*
*½ cup light corn syrup or golden syrup, such as Lyle's*
*3½ ounces white chocolate, broken into pieces*

Line a muffin pan with 12 paper cups.

In a bowl, combine the oats, Rice Krispies, exotic dried fruits, and pecans. Put the butter, syrup, and white chocolate into a saucepan and heat gently until melted. Stir into the dry ingredients until they are well coated.

Divide the mixture among the paper cups, pressing down lightly. Store in the fridge.

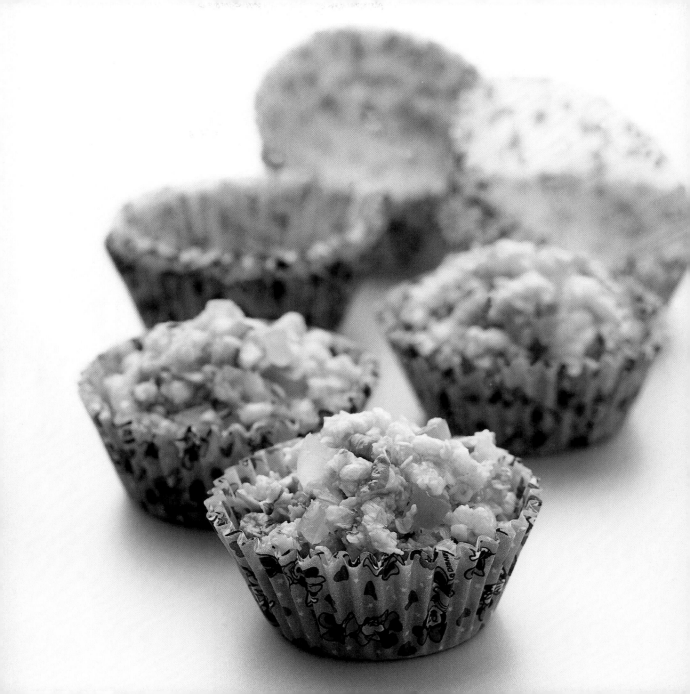

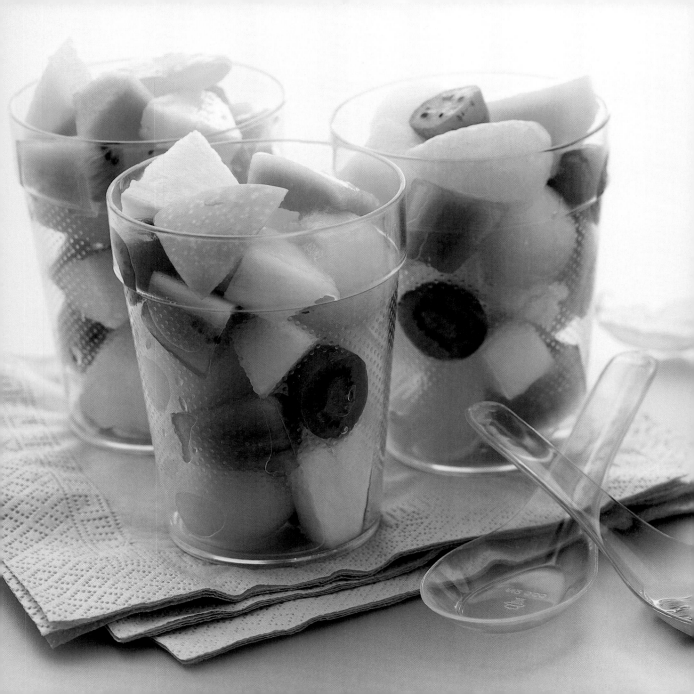

# great ways with fruit

**Every packed lunch should contain some fresh fruit. As well as containing lots of healthy nutrients, all fruit, including dried fruit, is a source of instant energy, as its natural sugars are easily digested.**

## fruit wedges

Children like to hold wedges of fruit, so try cutting a variety of fruits into wedges and packing them in a plastic container with a lid. For added interest, give a combination of fruit—pineapple, papaya, and mango go particularly well together. Fruits that make good wedges are:

- *Mango* • *Pineapple* • *Melon* • *Orange* • *Peach*
  • *Papaya* • *Pear* • *Kiwifruit*

## balls of fruit

Scoop out balls from different-colored melons—for example, honeydew and cantaloupe—and add some red and white grapes. Watermelon works well, too.

## fruit on a stick

Thread a selection of fruits onto a thin straw. You can use a mixture of fresh and dried fruits—for example, kiwifruit, pineapple, grapes, strawberries, and dried apricots.

**LUNCH BOX LOWDOWN**
Most children will leave food that takes a lot of effort to eat, as they want a quick refueling stop, leaving maximum time for the playground. So, give clementines or tangerines, peeled and covered with plastic wrap, or cut a kiwifruit in half and let your child scoop out the flesh with a teaspoon. Make sure he can easily open his lunch box and drinks container.

# quick and easy fruit salad

You can make delicious fruit salads using any fruits that are in season. Peel and pit the fruit if necessary. I leave the skin on fruits like apples, plums, and peaches, as most of the vitamins lie just under the skin. Cut the fruit into bite-size chunks and mix with your chosen sauce. The sauce adds flavor and stops the fruit from discoloring.

▽ **Makes 1 portion**
*Fruit salad*
*Cantaloupe and honeydew melon balls*
*1 kiwifruit, peeled and cut into chunks*
*½ mango, peeled and cut into chunks*
*1 thick slice pineapple, cut into chunks*
*1 clementine or tangerine, divided into segments*

*Orange and lemon sauce*
*2 tablespoons freshly squeezed orange juice*
*1 tablespoon lemon juice*
*2 teaspoons superfine sugar*
*seeds of 1 passion fruit (optional)*

To make the orange and lemon sauce, mix the juices and stir in the sugar until dissolved. Add the passion fruit seeds (if using).

# ruby red fruit salad

This is my favorite fruit salad. It has a wonderful flavor due to the rose water (available from large supermarkets), and the pomegranate adds a crunchy texture that complements the berry fruits beautifully. This will keep in the fridge for several days.

▽ **Makes 3 portions**
*2 large red plums, halved and pitted*
*1 large ripe peach, halved and pitted*
*1½ tablespoons unsalted butter*
*1½ to 2 tablespoons superfine sugar (to taste)*
*1 tablespoon rose water or orange flower water*
*  (you can also use plain water)*
*½ cup raspberries*
*½ cup blueberries*
*½ cup blackberries*
*seeds of 1 small pomegranate*

Cut each plum into eight pieces and cut the peach into twelve pieces. Melt the butter in a large frying pan and add the plums and the peach. Cook for 2 minutes, then turn over and sprinkle with the sugar. Cook for a further 2 to 3 minutes, then pour in the rose water. Gently stir in the remaining fruits, including the pomegranate seeds, and heat through for about 1 minute. Allow to cool.

# fresh berries with summer-fruit coulis and yogurt

Berry fruits are rich in vitamin C, which is a powerful antioxidant needed for growth and healthy skin, and it also helps the body absorb iron. We can't store vitamin C in our bodies, so we need to eat vitamin C–rich foods every day. As a variation on this recipe, mix the fresh berries with the summer-fruit coulis and leave out the yogurt.

▽ **Makes 1 portion**
*Summer-fruit coulis*
*³/₄ cup mixed frozen summer fruits, such as strawberries, raspberries, blueberries, blackberries, cherries, and red currants*
*2 tablespoons superfine sugar*

*one 6-ounce container Greek-style yogurt*
*³/₄ cup mixed fresh berries, such as blueberries, raspberries, and strawberries*

To make the coulis, put the frozen fruit and the sugar into a saucepan. Bring to a boil and simmer for 5 minutes. Puree in a blender, strain, and transfer to a container with a tight-fitting lid.

Spoon the yogurt into a plastic container with the mixed fresh berries. Leave ready for your child to pour the coulis over the yogurt and berries at lunchtime.

# apple, plum, and blackberry compote

There are some delicious fruit compotes to be made—try this mixed-fruit version. Fuji or Granny Smith apples cooked with a little sugar until tender are also delicious. Compotes tend to taste best when made with slightly tart fruit.

▽ **Makes 4 to 5 portions**
*1 large cooking apple, such as McIntosh or Macoun, peeled, cored, and chopped*
*4 plums, halved, pitted, and sliced*
*¹/₃ cup superfine sugar*
*1 vanilla bean or a pinch of ground cinnamon*
*1 cup blackberries*

Place the apple, plums, and sugar in a saucepan. Split the vanilla bean, scrape out the seeds, and add these and the bean (or the cinnamon, if preferred) to the pan. Cover with a lid and cook for about 15 minutes. Add the blackberries, cover, and simmer for a further 5 minutes. Remove the vanilla bean (if using), leave the fruit to cool, then put the compote in the fridge to chill.

# fruit smoothies

**Giving your children something nutritious to drink, like a smoothie, is a good way to ensure that they get the vitamins and minerals they need. It can be fun for children to make smoothies themselves.**

## mango, coconut, and pineapple

◯ **Makes 2 glasses**
$1/2$ cup canned coconut milk
$1/2$ mango, peeled and cut into chunks
$1/2$ cup pineapple juice
$1/2$ cup peach yogurt drink
1 small banana, cut into chunks

Mix together all the ingredients and puree in a blender until beautifully smooth. Pour into a glass to serve.

## sunshine smoothie

◯ **Makes 1 glass**
1 medium banana, cut into chunks
handful of mango chunks
1 teaspoon honey
$1/2$ cup pineapple juice
$1/4$ cup orange juice

Put the banana, mango, and honey into a blender and whiz for 1 to 2 minutes until smooth. Add the pineapple and orange juices and whiz again until frothy. Pour into a glass to serve.

## strawberries and cream

◯ **Makes 1 glass**
1 medium banana, cut into chunks
handful of strawberries, hulled and halved
3 tablespoons strawberry yogurt drink
$1/4$ cup cream soda

Put the banana, strawberries, and yogurt into a blender and blend for 1 to 2 minutes until smooth. Add the cream soda and whiz again until frothy. Pour into a glass to serve.

## peach melba

◯ **Makes 2 glasses**
$1/4$ cup fresh raspberries
one 8-ounce can sliced peaches
1 cup raspberry yogurt drink
$1/4$ cup milk
1 tablespoon confectioners' sugar (or to taste)

Puree together the raspberries and peach slices and push through a sieve to remove the seeds. Using a hand blender, blend the fruits with the yogurt, milk, and sugar until smooth.

*(see photograph on pages 96–97)*

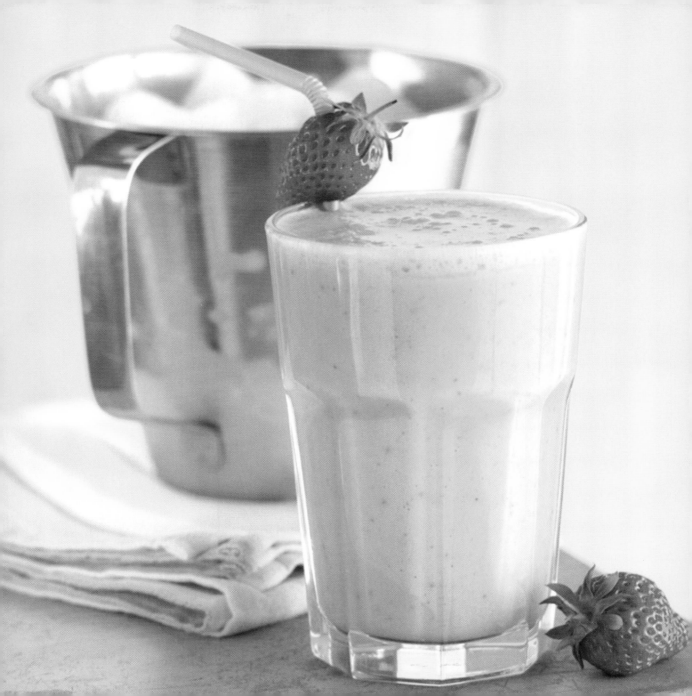

# ice pops

**If there is one food that no child can resist, it's an ice pop; however, most ready-made pops are full of artificial flavoring and coloring. So, why not make your own using fresh fruit, fruit juice, and yogurt?**

## tropical fruit pops

You will need four ice pop molds.

▽ **Makes 4 large pops**
*1 large mango, peeled and diced*
*¾ cup tropical fruit juice*
*3 tablespoons confectioners' sugar*
*1 tablespoon lemon juice*

Blend the ingredients together until smooth. Pour into ice pop molds and freeze until solid.

---

### LUNCH BOX LOWDOWN

If you include a plum, nectarine, or other squishy food in your child's lunch box, wrap it in several layers of kitchen towel, then put it in a plastic bag.

---

## strawberry sorbet pops

Strawberries contain higher levels of vitamin C than any other berries, so they are a great fruit to give your child. You will need four ice pop molds.

▽ **Makes 4 ice pops**
*2 tablespoons superfine sugar*
*2 tablespoons water*
*1½ cups strawberries, hulled and halved*
*2 tablespoons freshly squeezed orange juice*

Put the sugar and water into a saucepan and boil until syrupy (about 3 minutes). Allow to cool. Puree the strawberries with an electric hand blender and mix with the cooled syrup and the orange juice. Pour into ice pop molds and freeze until solid.

## strawberry and orange pops

By freezing in two stages, you can make wonderful two-color ice pops. You can achieve this using fruit juice or smoothies, or follow the method below. You could use other juices, such as tropical fruit juice, instead of orange. You will need four ice pop molds.

▽ **Makes 4 small two-color pops**
*¼ cup strawberry sorbet, softened*
*1¼ cups orange juice*

Pour the strawberry sorbet into the molds so that they are each about one-third full. Freeze for 1½ to 2 hours until frozen, then fill to the top with the orange juice and return to the freezer.

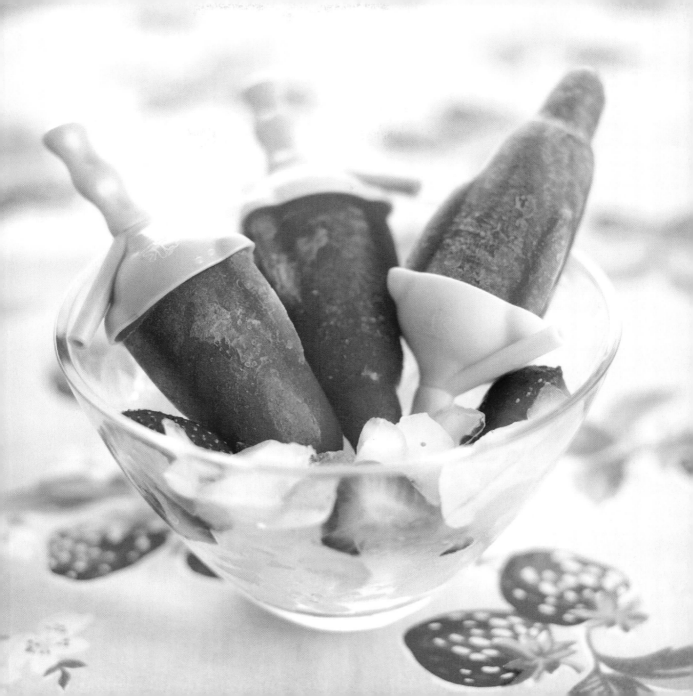

# index

## acknowledgments

For the creation of this book, my thanks go to Ian Jackson and Nick Eddison at Eddison Sadd and Grace Cheetham at Ebury. Many thanks to Dave King and William Lingwood for the beautiful photography.

I would like to thank Caroline Stearns for helping me create some of the delicious recipes in this new edition; Marina Magpoc; Letty Catada; Nadine Wickenden; at Simon & Schuster, Judith Curr, Greer Hendricks, Sarah Walsh, Sybil Pincus, Virginia McRae, Maralee Youngs, Annette Corkey, Christine Saunders, Kathleen Schmidt, and Gary Urda; and my children, Nicholas, Lara, and Scarlett, and all their friends for trying out my new recipes.

## about the author

**Annabel Karmel** is a leading author on cooking for children. After the tragic loss of her first child, who died of a rare viral disease at just three months, she wrote her first book, *The Healthy Baby Meal Planner*, which is now an international bestseller. Annabel has written fourteen more bestselling books on feeding children, including *Top 100 Baby Purees*, *Favorite Family Meals*, *First Meals*, and *Complete Party Planner*. The mother of three, she is an expert at creating tasty and nutritious meals that children like to eat without the need for parents to spend hours in the kitchen. Annabel writes regularly for national newspapers and is a familiar face on British television as an expert on children's nutritional issues. She travels frequently to the United States, where her books on feeding babies and young children are very popular, and has appeared on the *Today* show, *The Early Show*, and *The View*. Annabel has recently launched a Make Your Own line of equipment and foods to help parents prepare fresh baby food, and she has her own line of refrigerated ready-to-eat meals for children called Eat Fussy. She was awarded an MBE (Member of the British Empire) by the Queen in 2006 for her work in the field of child nutrition. For more information, visit www.annabelkarmel.com.